MAKING SENSE of the
ECG
Cases for Self Assessment

8/10/19

13/1/20

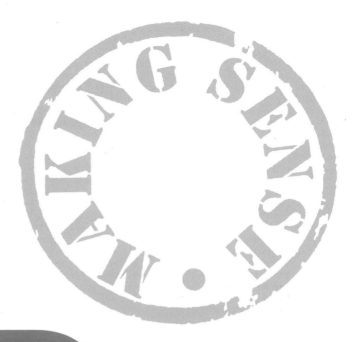

MAKING SENSE of the
ECG
Cases for Self Assessment

Second edition

Andrew R Houghton
Consultant Cardiologist, Grantham and District Hospital
and Visiting Fellow, University of Lincoln,
Lincolnshire, UK

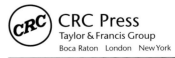

CRC Press
Taylor & Francis Group
Boca Raton   London   New York

CRC Press is an imprint of the
Taylor & Francis Group, an **informa** business

CRC Press
Taylor & Francis Group
6000 Broken Sound Parkway NW, Suite 300
Boca Raton, FL 33487-2742

© 2014 by Taylor & Francis Group, LLC
CRC Press is an imprint of Taylor & Francis Group, an Informa business

No claim to original U.S. Government works

Printed on acid-free paper
Version Date: 20140313

Printed and bound in India by Replika Press Pvt. Ltd.

International Standard Book Number-13: 978-1-4441-8184-5 (Paperback)

**Visit the Taylor & Francis Web site at
http://www.taylorandfrancis.com**

**and the CRC Press Web site at
http://www.crcpress.com**

To Kathryn and Caroline

Contents

Preface to the second edition

If you have already read our book *Making Sense of the ECG* fourth edition you may now be keen to put your knowledge to the test. In this companion volume, *Making Sense of the ECG: Cases for Self-Assessment* second edition, you can test your skills in ECG interpretation with 70 individual clinical cases.

This book is simple to use. Each of the cases begins with an ECG, an illustrative clinical scenario (to place the ECG in an appropriate context), and a number of questions. On turning the page, you will find the answers to the questions together with a detailed analysis of the ECG. This is followed by a general commentary on the ECG and the clinical case, and suggestions for further reading. The ECG cases are presented in order of increasing difficulty and we are certain that whatever your experience in ECG interpretation, you will find cases to challenge your skills.

We have revised and fully updated the text for this new edition and provided up-to-date references to relevant papers and guidelines. Several cases have been replaced with new examples. All the cross-references to our new companion volume, *Making Sense of the ECG* fourth edition, have been updated.

Once again, we are grateful to everyone who has taken the time to comment on the text and to provide us with ECGs from their collections. Finally, we would like to thank all the staff at CRC Press who have contributed to the success of the *Making Sense* series of books.

Andrew R Houghton
David Gray
2014

Acknowledgements

We would like to thank everyone who gave us suggestions and constructive criticism while we have prepared each edition of *Making Sense of the ECG: Cases for Self-Assessment*. We are particularly grateful to the following for their invaluable comments on the text and for allowing us to use ECGs from their collections:

Mookhter Ajij

Khin Maung Aye

Stephanie Baker

Michael Bamber

Muneer Ahmad Bhat

Gabriella Captur

Andrea Charman

Nigel Dewey

Matthew Donnelly

Ian Ferrer

Catherine Goult

Lawrence Green

Mahesh Harishchandra

Michael Holmes

Safiy Karim

Dave Kendall

Jeffrey Khoo

Daniel Law

Diane Lunn

Iain Lyburn

Sonia Lyburn

Martin Melville

Cara Mercer

Yuji Murakawa

Francis Murgatroyd

V B S Naidu

Vicky Nelmes

Claire Poole

George B Pradhan

Jane Robinson

Catherine Scott

Penelope R. Sensky

Neville Smith

Gary Spiers

Andrew Staniforth

Andrew Stein

Robin Touquet

Upul Wijayawardhana

Bernadette Williamson

Finally, we would also like to express our gratitude to Dr Joanna Koster and the rest of the publishing team at CRC Press for their encouragement, guidance and support during this project.

Normal values

Full Blood Count (FBC)

Hb	13.5–16.9 g/dL (male)
	11.5–14.8 g/dL (female)
White cell count (WCC)	$4.5–13.0 \times 10^9$/L
Platelets	$150–400 \times 10^9$/L

Urea and Electrolytes (U&E)

Na	136–145 mmol/L
K	3.5–5.1 mmol/L
Urea	3.2–7.4 mmol/L (male)
	2.5–6.7 mmol/L (female)
Creatinine	53–115 mmol/L

CASE 1

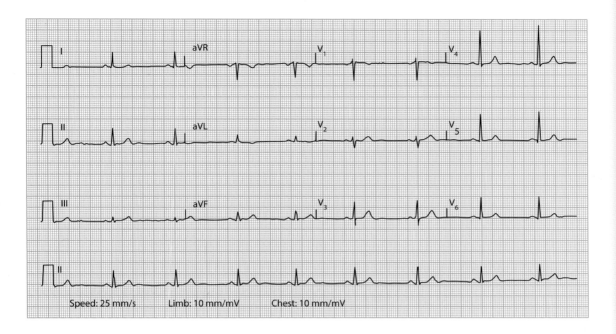

Speed: 25 mm/s   Limb: 10 mm/mV   Chest: 10 mm/mV

CLINICAL SCENARIO

Male, aged 28 years.

Presenting complaint
Asymptomatic fitness instructor. This screening ECG was performed at a 'well man' medical check-up.

History of presenting complaint
Nil – the patient is asymptomatic.

Past medical history
Appendicectomy (aged 17 years).

Examination
Athletic build.
Pulse: 50/min, regular.
Blood pressure: 128/80.
JVP: not elevated.
Heart sounds: normal.
Chest auscultation: unremarkable.
No peripheral oedema.
Old appendicectomy scar noted in right iliac fossa.

Investigations
FBC: Hb 14.8, WCC 6.2, platelets 229.
U&E: Na 140, K 4.4, urea 3.7, creatinine 78.
Thyroid function: normal.
Chest X-ray: normal heart size, clear lung fields.

QUESTIONS

1. What does this ECG show?
2. How did you calculate the heart rate?
3. Is the heart rate normal?
4. Is any further action required?

ECG ANALYSIS

Rate	50/min
Rhythm	Sinus bradycardia
QRS axis	Normal (+42°)
P waves	Normal
PR interval	Normal (160 ms)
QRS duration	Normal (76 ms)
T waves	Normal
QTc interval	Normal (407 ms)

Additional comments

There is a very slight variation in heart rate on the ECG – the distance between consecutive QRS complexes (the R-R interval) varies slightly. This is not unusual, and results from a slight variation in heart rate with respiration.

ANSWERS

1. This ECG shows mild sinus bradycardia, but is otherwise normal.
2. There are several ways to calculate heart rate:
   - At a standard paper speed of 25 mm/s, there will be 300 large squares for every minute of ECG recording. You can therefore count the number of large squares between two consecutive QRS complexes – in this example, there are 6 – and then divide this number into 300 (i.e. 300/6). This gives a heart rate of 50/min.
   - An alternative, and slightly more accurate, method is to count small squares rather than big ones. For this method, you need to remember than a 1-min ECG recording covers 1500 small squares. Count the number of small squares between two consecutive QRS complexes, and divide it into 1500.
   - The above methods are best used when the rhythm is regular. If the rhythm is irregular (e.g. atrial fibrillation) it is better to count the total number of QRS complexes along a strip 30 large squares in length. A strip of 30 large squares is equivalent to 6 s of recording (at a paper speed of 25 mm/s). You can therefore count the number of QRS complexes in 30 large squares, and then multiply this number by 10 to give the number of QRS complexes per minute.
3. Generally speaking, bradycardia is defined as a heart rate below 60/min. However, it is always important to assess clinical data in the context of the patient. This is a young patient, with an athletic background, and so a relatively slow resting heart rate is not unusual. In this clinical context, the mild sinus bradycardia is not of concern.
4. No – the patient can be reassured that the ECG is normal.

COMMENTARY

- One of the most important principles of ECG interpretation, and indeed in interpreting any test result, is to place things in their clinical context. Although the 'normal range' for the heart rate in sinus rhythm is 60–100/min, a rate between 50–60/min is seldom of any significance or clinical consequence. If a patient is athletic it is not unusual to have a mild resting bradycardia and it is important not to diagnose this as pathological.

- Whenever you interpret an ECG, it is important to begin by asking 'How is the patient?' This will give you the clinical context you require to make a correct assessment. Similarly, if you make an ECG recording, it is good practice to make a note of the clinical context at the top of the ECG, along with the patient's identification details and the date/time of the recording. This can take the form of a brief sentence to say 'Patient complaining of palpitations', or 'Patient experiencing severe chest tightness', or just 'Routine ECG – patient asymptomatic'. This makes it much easier for you – and for others – to interpret the ECG when it is reviewed later on.

- A mild sinus bradycardia can also be the result of drug treatment (particularly beta blockers, digoxin, ivabradine or rate-limiting calcium channel blockers, such as verapamil). Don't forget about beta blocking eye drops, which can have systemic effects.

- The T wave inversion seen in lead aVR and in lead V1 is a normal finding.

Further reading

Making Sense of the ECG 4th edition: Heart rate, p 35; Sinus rhythm, p 53; Sinus bradycardia, p 54.

Meek S, Morri F. ABC of clinical electrocardiography: Introduction. I—Leads, rate, rhythm, and cardiac axis. *Br Med J* 2002; **324**: 415–8.

CASE 2

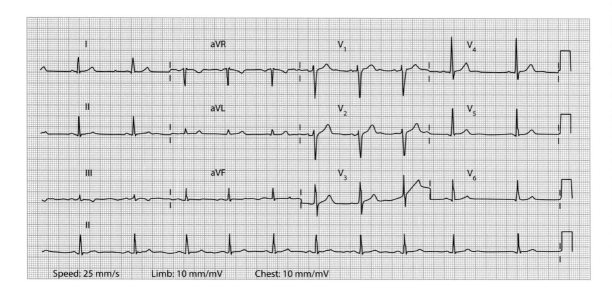

Speed: 25 mm/s   Limb: 10 mm/mV   Chest: 10 mm/mV

CLINICAL SCENARIO

Male, aged 27 years.

Presenting complaint
No cardiac symptoms but aware he has an 'abnormal ECG'.

History of presenting complaint
Patient had been scheduled for knee surgery and was seen by a nurse in the surgical preoperative assessment clinic. The nurse reported a slightly irregular pulse and requested an ECG. Subsequently the patient was referred to the cardiology clinic for a preoperative cardiac opinion.

Past medical history
Nil of note.

Examination
Pulse: 60/min, slightly irregular.
Blood pressure: 126/88.
JVP: not elevated.
Heart sounds: normal.
Chest auscultation: unremarkable.
No peripheral oedema.

Investigations
FBC: Hb 16.5, WCC 4.3, platelets 353.
U&E: Na 140, K 4.5, urea 4.4, creatinine 98.
Thyroid function: normal.
Chest X-ray: normal heart size, clear lung fields.

QUESTIONS

1. What does this ECG show?
2. What is the mechanism of this?
3. What is the likely cause?
4. What are the key issues in managing this patient?

ECG ANALYSIS

Rate	60/min
Rhythm	Sinus arrhythmia
QRS axis	Normal (+43°)
P waves	Normal
PR interval	Normal (160 ms)
QRS duration	Normal (100 ms)
T waves	Normal
QTc interval	Normal (400 ms)

ANSWERS

1. Every P wave is followed by a normal QRS complex, but the heart rate varies. Observation of the patient confirms that this coincides with respiration, with the heart rate increasing on inspiration and decreasing on expiration. This is **sinus arrhythmia**.

2. There is variation in the heart rate in response to respiration, increasing reflexly during inspiration (due to increased venous return to the heart) and decreasing during expiration.

3. This is a normal physiological response. The exact mechanism of sinus arrhythmia has been the subject of investigation and debate for many years. There is some evidence that the respiratory variation in heart rate is mediated via carotid baroreceptors and/or cardiopulmonary receptors. Others suggest a central mechanism. (Heart rate is normally controlled by centres in the medulla oblongata. One centre, the nucleus ambiguus, provides parasympathetic input to the heart via the vagus nerve, affecting the sinoatrial node. Inspiration signals the nucleus accumbens to inhibit the vagus nerve, increasing heart rate, while expiration increases vagal activity and reduces heart rate.)

4. No action is needed. Reassure the patient (and the pre-assessment clinic staff) that sinus arrhythmia is a normal finding.

COMMENTARY

- Sinus arrhythmia is of no pathological consequence. Sinus arrhythmia is most often seen in the young and much less commonly in those over the age of 40 years.
- Normally, the heart rate in sinus rhythm changes very little at rest. In sinus arrhythmia, the slight variation in cycling usually exceeds 120 ms between the longest and the shortest cycle (cycle length is equal to the interval between successive R waves, the RR interval).
- Sinus arrhythmia may be aggravated by any factor that increases vagal tone.

Further reading

Making Sense of the ECG 4th edition: Sinus arrhythmia, p 54; Is the ventricular rhythm regular or irregular?, p 47.

Piepoli M, Sleight P, Leuzzi, S *et al.* Origin of respiratory sinus arrhythmia in conscious humans. An important role for arterial carotid baroreceptors. *Circulation* 1997; **95**: 1813–21.

CASE 3

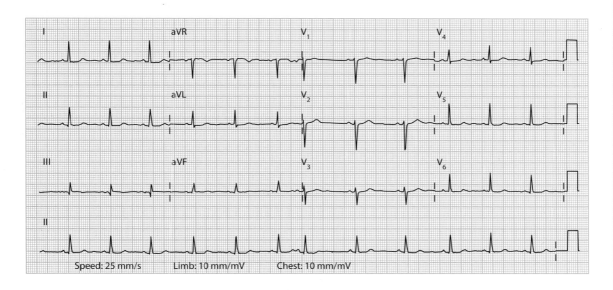

Speed: 25 mm/s   Limb: 10 mm/mV   Chest: 10 mm/mV

CLINICAL SCENARIO

Female, aged 36 years.

Presenting complaint
Palpitations.

History of presenting complaint
Six-month history of 'missed beats' occurring at rest, particularly when lying quietly in bed. Symptoms are more troublesome after drinking coffee.

Past medical history
Nil.

Examination
Pulse: 72/min, regular with occasional premature beat.
Blood pressure: 118/76.
JVP: not elevated.
Heart sounds: normal.
Chest auscultation: unremarkable.
No peripheral oedema.

Investigations
FBC: Hb 13.8, WCC 5.7, platelets 240.
U&E: Na 141, K 4.3, urea 2.8, creatinine 68.
Thyroid function: normal.

QUESTIONS

1. What does this ECG show?
2. What advice would you offer?
3. Is any drug treatment required?

ECG ANALYSIS

Rate	72/min
Rhythm	Sinus rhythm with an atrial ectopic beat
QRS axis	Normal (+27°)
P waves	Present
PR interval	Normal (120 ms)
QRS duration	Normal (70 ms)
T waves	Normal
QTc interval	Normal (416 ms)

Additional comments

The P wave associated with the atrial ectopic beat is visible just towards the end of the preceding T wave.

ANSWERS

1. This ECG shows normal sinus rhythm with a single **atrial ectopic beat** (the seventh beat along the rhythm strip).
2. The caffeine in coffee and in some cola drinks can be a trigger for atrial ectopic beats, and so advise the patient to switch to decaffeinated alternatives. Other cardiac stimulants (such as alcohol and nicotine) can also act as triggers and should be moderated or avoided as appropriate.
3. Drug treatment is seldom required unless the atrial ectopic beats cause particularly troublesome symptoms.

COMMENTARY

- Atrial ectopic beats are also known as atrial extrasystoles, atrial premature complexes (APCs), atrial premature beats (APBs) or premature atrial contractions (PACs). Atrial ectopic beats occur earlier than expected (in contrast with escape beats, which occur later than expected).
- Atrial ectopic beats can arise from any part of the atria, and the shape of the P wave depends upon where in the atria the ectopic has arisen from. In this patient's ECG, the P wave of the atrial ectopic beat has a shape very similar to the P wave of a normal sinus beat, suggesting an ectopic focus near to the sinoatrial node. In contrast, atrial ectopic beats that arise from low down in the atria, near the atrioventricular node, will have P waves that are inverted in the inferior leads but upright in lead aVR. This is because the wave of depolarization will predominantly move upwards in the atria, rather than downwards from the sinoatrial node. The P wave may also appear very close to, or overlap with, the QRS complex, as a focus of depolarization near the atrioventricular node will reach the ventricles more quickly than one that has to travel from the sinoatrial node.
- Avoidance of triggers such as caffeine, alcohol and nicotine is often sufficient to reduce the frequency of atrial ectopic beats. They are generally benign, and so drug treatment is not usually needed unless the associated sensation of palpitations is very frequent and troublesome. If treatment is required, beta blockers can be effective in suppressing atrial ectopic activity.

Further reading

Making Sense of the ECG 4th edition: Atrial ectopic beats, p 58.

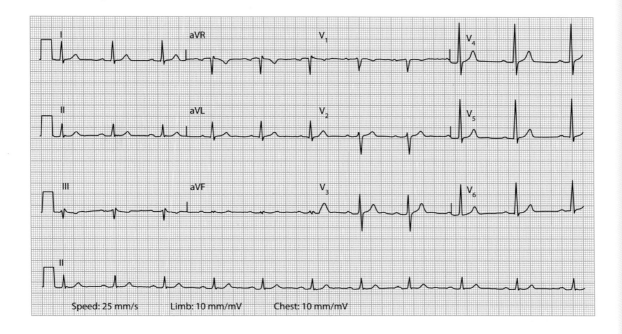

Speed: 25 mm/s   Limb: 10 mm/mV   Chest: 10 mm/mV

CLINICAL SCENARIO

Female, aged 73 years.

Presenting complaint
Asymptomatic.

History of presenting complaint
Patient had recently moved house. She saw her new family doctor for a routine health check which included an ECG. Automated print-out reported 'Abnormal ECG'.

Past medical history
Mild hypertension.
Diet-controlled diabetes mellitus.
Osteoarthritis and bilateral hip replacements.

Examination
Pulse: 66/min, regular.
Blood pressure: 152/98.
JVP: not elevated.
Heart sounds: normal.
Chest auscultation: unremarkable.
No peripheral oedema.

Investigations
FBC: Hb 12.4, WCC 6.7, platelets 296.
U&E: Na 134, K 3.8, urea 5.1, creatinine 99.
Chest X-ray: normal heart size, clear lung fields.
Echocardiogram: Trivial mitral regurgitation into a nondilated left atrium. Normal left ventricular function.

QUESTIONS

1. What does this ECG show?
2. What is the mechanism of this?
3. What are the likely causes?
4. What are the key issues in managing this patient?

ECG ANALYSIS

Rate	66/min
Rhythm	Sinus rhythm
QRS axis	Normal (+15°)
P waves	Normal
PR interval	Prolonged (240 ms)
QRS duration	Normal (100 ms)
T waves	Normal
QTc interval	Normal (420 ms)

ANSWERS

1. The PR interval (which is measured from the start of the P wave to the start of the QRS complex) is greater than 200 ms, so conduction through the atrioventricular node is delayed; this delay is constant for each cardiac cycle. This is **first-degree atrioventricular block** ('first-degree heart block').

2. First-degree atrioventricular block is caused by delayed conduction of the atrial impulse to the ventricles through the atrioventricular node.

3. First-degree atrioventricular block can be a feature of ischaemic heart disease, hyperkalaemia or hypokalaemia, acute rheumatic myocarditis, Lyme disease and drugs such as beta blockers, rate-limiting calcium-channel blockers and digoxin. It can also be a normal physiological finding, particularly in young people with high vagal tone (e.g. during sleep).

4. First-degree atrioventricular block does not cause symptoms in its own right and does not usually require any specific intervention.

COMMENTARY

- First-degree atrioventricular block is asymptomatic and no action is indicated. It rarely progresses to second- or third-degree atrioventricular block. It should however raise the possibility of one of the diagnoses listed above (which may require treatment in its own right).
- First-degree atrioventricular block is not an indication for pacing.

Further reading

Making Sense of the ECG 4th edition: First-degree atrioventricular block, p 94; Is the PR interval more than 0.2s long?, p 130.

CASE 5

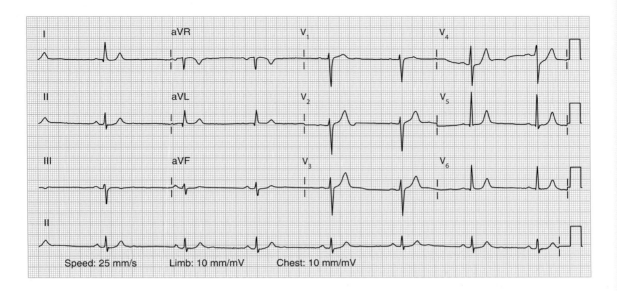

Speed: 25 mm/s   Limb: 10 mm/mV   Chest: 10 mm/mV

CLINICAL SCENARIO

Male, aged 66 years.

Presenting complaint
Fatigue.

History of presenting complaint
The patient was diagnosed with hypertension 6 weeks ago and was commenced on treatment. Since that time he has felt tired and has noticed a reduction in his exercise capacity.

Past medical history
Hypertension, treated with atenolol 50 mg once daily.

Examination
Pulse: 42/min, regular.
Blood pressure: 156/94.
JVP: not elevated.
Heart sounds: normal.
Chest auscultation: unremarkable.
No peripheral oedema.

Investigations
FBC: Hb 13.8, WCC 7.6, platelets 313.
U&E: Na 138, K 4.2, urea 5.2, creatinine 98.

QUESTIONS

1. What rhythm is seen on this ECG?
2. What investigations would be appropriate?
3. What treatment is needed?
4. Is a pacemaker required?

ECG ANALYSIS

Rate	42/min
Rhythm	Sinus bradycardia
QRS axis	Normal (+1°)
P waves	Normal
PR interval	Normal (195 ms)
QRS duration	Normal (100 ms)
T waves	Normal
QTc interval	Normal (368 ms)

ANSWERS

1. Sinus bradycardia, with a heart rate of 42/min.
2. In addition to the FBC and U&E listed, it would be appropriate to do thyroid function tests (to exclude hypothyroidism). An echocardiogram would determine whether left ventricular dysfunction is contributing to the patient's fatigue.
3. A reduction in the dose of the beta blocker, and possibly its complete withdrawal. Any reductions in beta blocker dose must be undertaken gradually to reduce the risk of 'rebound' tachycardia or hypertension.
4. A pacemaker is unlikely to be necessary – the clinical history makes it likely that the fatigue and bradycardia resulted from the recent introduction of a beta blocker, so the patient's fatigue should resolve on withdrawal of this.

COMMENTARY

- Sinus bradycardia can be a normal finding in athletic individuals and also in most people during sleep.

- Always looks for correctable causes such as drug treatment (particularly beta blockers, digoxin, ivabradine or rate-limiting calcium channel blockers, such as verapamil). Do not forget about beta blocking eye drops, which can have systemic effects. Other causes include hypothyroidism, hypothermia, myocardial ischaemia and infarction, raised intracranial pressure (look for the combination of falling pulse and rising blood pressure), uraemia, obstructive jaundice and electrolyte abnormalities.

- Beta blockers are not recommended as first-line drugs for the management of hypertension, unless other indications exist, and so it would be appropriate to replace the beta blocker with an alternative drug in this case. A suitable choice for a hypertensive patient over the age of 55 years would be a calcium channel blocker.

- Permanent pacing is a treatment for symptomatic bradycardia, but it is essential to make sure that other correctable causes are identified and treated first – in this case, withdrawal of any negatively chronotropic drugs (those that slow the heart). Sometimes temporary transvenous pacing is required to support the patient, if he/she is severely symptomatic from their bradycardia, while any correctible causes are identified and treated.

Further reading

Making Sense of the ECG 4th edition: Sinus bradycardia, p 54; Indications for temporary pacing, p 210; Indications for permanent pacing, p 211.

National Institute for Health and Care Excellence. *Hypertension: clinical management of primary hypertension in adults.* Clinical guideline 34. London: NICE, 2011. Available at http://guidance.nice.org.uk/CG127

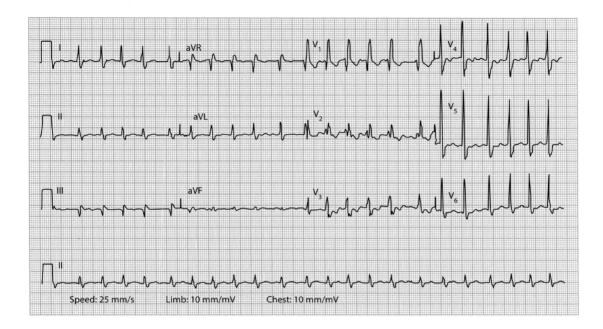

Speed: 25 mm/s   Limb: 10 mm/mV   Chest: 10 mm/mV

CLINICAL SCENARIO

Female, aged 79 years.

Presenting complaint
Palpitations and breathlessness.

History of presenting complaint
The patient had been well until 3 days ago. She noticed her heart beating faster when walking. She had also started to struggle when doing housework.

Past medical history
Ischaemic heart disease for 10 years. When she recently moved house and changed doctor, her usual beta blocker was omitted in error from the repeat prescription.

Examination
Pulse: 132/min, irregularly irregular.

Blood pressure: 120/70 approximately.
JVP: not seen (obese).
Heart sounds: normal.
Chest auscultation: fine basal crackles.
No peripheral oedema.

Investigations
FBC: Hb 11.7, WCC 5.6, platelets 310.
U&E: Na 141, K 4.3, urea 6.7, creatinine 124.
Thyroid function: normal.
Troponin I: negative.
Chest X-ray: mild cardiomegaly.
Echocardiogram: mild mitral regurgitation into nondilated left atrium. Left ventricular function moderately impaired (ejection fraction 43 per cent).

QUESTIONS

1. What does this ECG show?
2. What is the mechanism of this?
3. What are the likely causes?
4. What are the key issues in managing this patient?

ECG ANALYSIS

Rate	132/min
Rhythm	Atrial fibrillation
QRS axis	Normal (−4°)
P waves	Absent
PR interval	N/A
QRS duration	Prolonged (140 ms)
T waves	Inverted (leads V1–V4)
QTc interval	Mildly prolonged (474 ms)

Additional comments

There is a right bundle branch block (RBBB), which accounts for the T wave inversion.

ANSWERS

1. The irregularly irregular rhythm with no discernible P waves means that this is **atrial fibrillation** AF (with a fast ventricular response). There is also RBBB.
2. The basis of AF is rapid, chaotic depolarization occurring throughout the atria as a consequence of multiple 'wavelets' of activation. No P waves are seen and the ECG baseline consists of low-amplitude oscillations (fibrillation or 'f' waves). Although around 400–600 impulses reach the AV node every minute, only some will be transmitted to the ventricles. The ventricular rate is typically fast (100–180/min), although the rate can be normal or even slow. Transmission of the atrial impulses through the AV node is erratic, making the ventricular (QRS complex) rhythm 'irregularly irregular'.
3. There are many possible causes of AF. These include hypertension, ischaemic heart disease, valvular heart disease, cardiomyopathies, myocarditis, atrial septal defect and other congenital heart disease, hyperthyroidism, alcohol, pulmonary embolism, pneumonia and cardiac surgery. AF can also be idiopathic ('lone atrial fibrillation').
4. Patients with AF require a careful assessment to identify (and treat) the underlying cause. This includes a thorough history and examination, 12-lead ECG and blood tests to check electrolytes and renal function, thyroid function tests and a full blood count. Echocardiography is used to screen for structural heart disease. Risk stratify the patient with regard to thromboembolic (and bleeding) risk and anticoagulate as appropriate. Decide whether attempting to restore (and maintain) sinus rhythm would be appropriate, or whether to accept AF and pursue a rate control strategy. Where appropriate, investigations for coronary artery disease may also be required. Where necessary, ventricular rate control can be achieved with beta blockers, rate-limiting calcium channel blockers, digoxin or, if other alternatives cannot be used, amiodarone.

COMMENTARY

- AF is common (the commonest sustained arrhythmia) and its prevalence increases with age.
- AF may be:
  - **first-diagnosed** – namely, patients presenting in atrial fibrillation for the first time
  - **paroxysmal** – self-terminating episodes, typically lasting <48h although they can last up to 7 days
  - **persistent** – an episode of continuous atrial fibrillation lasting >7 days or requiring cardioversion
  - **long-standing persistent** – where AF has been present for at least one year, but there is still an aim to restore sinus rhythm
  - **permanent** – continuous AF where the arrhythmia is 'accepted' and there is no plan to restore sinus rhythm.
- AF may be asymptomatic, but can be accompanied by awareness of an irregular heartbeat, dyspnoea, fatigue, dizziness and syncope.
- The presence of AF increases a patient's stroke risk five-fold, and one in five strokes occurs as a result of AF. Strokes that occur in AF are more likely to be disabling or fatal.
- For patients with valvular AF (including rheumatic valve disease and prosthetic valves), anticoagulation with warfarin is recommended for all, unless there are contraindications.

- For those with non-valvular AF, antithrombotic therapy is recommended for all, except in those patients who are at low risk (aged <65 years and lone AF), or with contraindications. Where antithrombotic therapy is indicated, this should be with warfarin or one of the novel oral anticoagulants, such as dabigatran. If patients refuse oral anticoagulants, antiplatelet therapy (using aspirin 75–100 mg plus clopidogrel 75 mg daily or, less effectively, aspirin 75–325 mg daily) may be considered as an alternative.

Further reading

Making Sense of the ECG 4th edition: Atrial fibrillation, p 59; Is the ventricular rhythm regular or irregular?, p 47.

Camm AJ, Kirchhof P, Lip GY *et al.* Guidelines for the management of atrial fibrillation: the Task Force for the Management of Atrial Fibrillation of the European Society of Cardiology (ESC). *Europace* 2010; **12**: 1360–420.

Camm AJ, Lip GYH, De Caterina R *et al.* 2012 focused update of the ESC guidelines for the management of atrial fibrillation. *Eur Heart J* 2012; **33**: 2719–47.

CASE 7

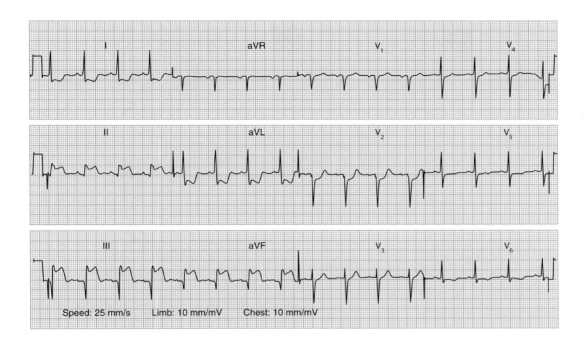

Speed: 25 mm/s   Limb: 10 mm/mV   Chest: 10 mm/mV

CLINICAL SCENARIO

Male, aged 71 years.

Presenting complaint
Crushing central chest pain.

History of presenting complaint
Two-hour history of crushing central chest pain, which awoke the patient at 4:00 am. The pain radiates to the left arm and is associated with breathlessness, nausea and sweating.

Past medical history
Angina diagnosed 1 year ago.
Hypertension diagnosed 6 years ago.
Active cigarette smoker (48 pack-year smoking history).

Examination
Clammy, in pain.
Pulse: 85/min, regular.
Blood pressure: 148/82.
JVP: not elevated.
Heart sounds: normal.
Chest auscultation: unremarkable.
No peripheral oedema.

Investigations
FBC: Hb 13.8, WCC 10.2, platelets 349.
U&E: Na 138, K 4.2, urea 5.7, creatinine 98.
Troponin I: elevated at 1643 (after 6 h).
Chest X-ray: normal heart size, clear lung fields.
Echocardiogram: akinesia of inferior wall of left ventricle, overall ejection fraction 50 per cent.

QUESTIONS

1. What does this ECG show?
2. What other type of ECG recording should be performed? Why should this be done?
3. What treatment is indicated?
4. Should this ECG be repeated? When should it be repeated and why?

ECG ANALYSIS

Rate	85/min
Rhythm	Sinus rhythm
QRS axis	Normal (+10°)
P waves	Present
PR interval	Normal (154 ms)
QRS duration	Normal (92 ms)
T waves	Lateral T inversion
QTc interval	Normal (428 ms)

Additional comments

There is ST segment elevation in the inferior leads (II, III, aVF) with reciprocal ST/T wave changes in the lateral leads (I, aVL, V5–V6).

ANSWERS

1. This ECG shows an acute inferior ST segment elevation myocardial infarction (STEMI).
2. Another ECG should be performed immediately using right-sided chest leads (V1R–V6R) to look for evidence of right ventricular involvement in the inferior myocardial infarction.
3. Aspirin 300 mg orally (then 75 mg once daily), clopidogrel 300 mg orally (then 75 mg once daily), glyceryl trinitrate sublingually, pain relief (an opioid intravenously, plus an anti-emetic), oxygen if hypoxic. Prompt restoration of myocardial blood flow is required by primary percutaneous coronary intervention (PCI) or, if primary PCI is not available, thrombolysis.
4. Yes – if thrombolysis is used, the ECG must be repeated 90 min after the start of thrombolysis to determine whether coronary reperfusion has successfully been achieved. This is shown by resolution of the ST segment elevation by ≥50 per cent. In addition, whether primary PCI or thrombolysis is used, the ECG must be monitored throughout coronary reperfusion because of the risk of arrhythmias.

COMMENTARY

- An urgent ECG is required in any patient presenting with cardiac-sounding chest pain.

The presence of ST segment elevation signifies acute occlusion of a coronary artery and indicates a need for urgent restoration of coronary blood flow (reperfusion). This can be achieved with primary PCI or with thrombolysis. Time is of the essence – the longer reperfusion is delayed, the more myocardial necrosis will occur.

- The right ventricle is involved in 10–50 per cent of inferior ST segment elevation myocardial infarctions. It can be diagnosed by performing an ECG using right-sided chest leads (V1R–V6R) and looking for ST segment elevation in V4R. Right ventricular infarction is important to recognize because it can have significant haemodynamic consequences. It may lead to signs of right heart failure (raised jugular venous pressure and peripheral oedema). If these patients develop hypotension, this may be because of failure of the right ventricle to pump sufficient blood to the left ventricle. Thus, despite the signs of right heart failure, it may be necessary to give intravenous fluids to maintain left heart filling pressures. This is one situation in which haemodynamic monitoring with Swan–Ganz catheterization can prove helpful.
- A failure to achieve coronary reperfusion after thrombolysis may indicate the need to consider repeat thrombolysis or coronary angiography and 'rescue' PCI. If the ST segment elevation has not fallen by ≥50 per cent 2 h after the start of thrombolysis, there is an 80–85 per cent probability that normal coronary blood flow has not been restored.
- The differential diagnosis of ST segment elevation includes acute myocardial infarction, left ventricular aneurysm, Prinzmetal's (vaso-spastic) angina, pericarditis, high take-off, left bundle branch block and Brugada syndrome.

Further reading

Making Sense of the ECG 4th edition: Are the ST segments elevated? p 159; ST segment elevation myocardial infarction p 160; Why is right ventricular infarction important? p 165.

de Belder MA. Acute myocardial infarction: failed thrombolysis. *Heart* 2001; **81**: 104–12.

CASE 8

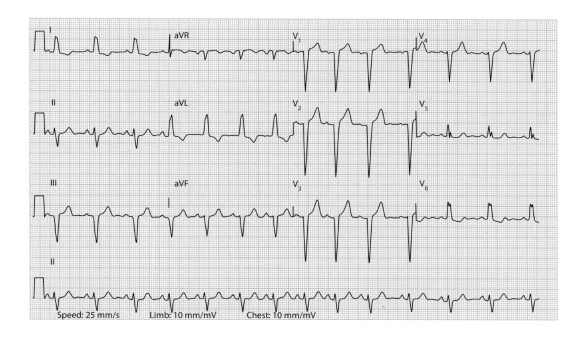

Speed: 25 mm/s   Limb: 10 mm/mV   Chest: 10 mm/mV

CLINICAL SCENARIO

Male, aged 80 years.

Presenting complaint
Exertional chest pain, usually when walking uphill in cold and windy weather.

History of presenting complaint
Had been referred to hospital a few years ago with symptoms of exertional chest pain and diagnosed with angina.

Past medical history
Hypertension – well controlled.
Mild chronic airways disease.
Type 2 diabetes mellitus.
Is scheduled for prostatectomy – this ECG was recorded at preoperative assessment clinic.

Examination
Pulse: 84/min.
Blood pressure: 148/96.
JVP: not elevated.
Heart sounds: normal.
Chest auscultation: unremarkable.
No peripheral oedema.

Investigations
FBC: Hb 12.7, WCC 6.4, platelets 400.
U&E: Na 142, K 3.9, urea 6.5, creatinine 144.
Chest X-ray: mild cardiomegaly, early pulmonary congestion.
Echocardiogram: moderately impaired left ventricular function (ejection fraction 42 per cent).

QUESTIONS

1. What does this ECG show?
2. What is the underlying mechanism?
3. What are the likely causes?
4. What are the key issues in managing this patient?

ECG ANALYSIS

Rate	84/min
Rhythm	Sinus rhythm
QRS axis	Left axis deviation (−51°)
P waves	Normal
PR interval	Normal (160 ms)
QRS duration	Prolonged (125 ms)
T waves	Inverted in leads I, aVL, V6
QTc interval	Mildly prolonged (460 ms)

ANSWERS

1. This ECG shows sinus rhythm with broadened and notched QRS complexes (QRS duration >120 ms), QS in lead V1 and a broad notched R wave in V6: this is **left bundle branch block** (LBBB).

2. LBBB results from a failure of conduction in the left bundle branch. The left ventricle must be activated indirectly via the right bundle branch, so the right ventricle is activated before the left ventricle. This lengthens the overall duration of ventricular depolarization and therefore broadens the QRS complexes (greater than 120 ms) and also distorts the QRS complexes. Repolarization is also abnormal, and ST segment depression and T wave inversion are frequently seen. LBBB may also be intermittent – especially in acute myocardial ischaemia. It may also occur with tachycardia (although rate-related bundle branch block more commonly causes right bundle branch block).

3. The causes of LBBB include ischaemic heart disease, cardiomyopathy, left ventricular hypertrophy (secondary to hypertension or aortic stenosis) and fibrosis of the conduction system.

4. The presence of LBBB is almost invariably pathological. Investigations are appropriate in the clinical context of chest pain, breathlessness and palpitations and also when LBBB is an incidental finding preoperatively. Echocardiography is useful in looking for cardiomyopathy, left ventricular hypertrophy and valve disease. Options to investigate for evidence of ischaemic heart disease include functional imaging (stress echocardiography, stress cardiac MRI or nuclear myocardial perfusion imaging) or anatomical imaging (CT or invasive coronary angiography).

COMMENTARY

- LBBB is commonly seen in the elderly. In the absence of symptoms or when perioperative risk assessment is not warranted, no investigations are necessary.

Further reading

Making Sense of the ECG 4th edition: Bundle branch block, p 153; Left bundle branch block, p 97.

Francia P, Balla C, Paneni F *et al.* Left bundle-branch block – pathophysiology, prognosis, and clinical management. *Clin Cardiol* 2007; **30**: 110–5.

CASE 9

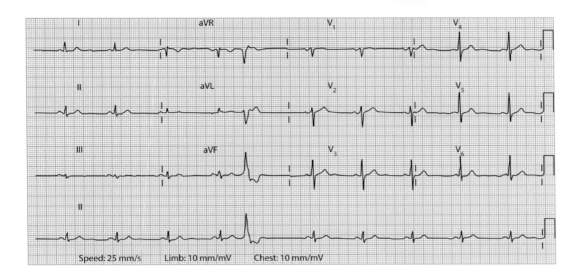

| | | Speed: 25 mm/s | Limb: 10 mm/mV | Chest: 10 mm/mV |

CLINICAL SCENARIO

Male, aged 61 years.

Presenting complaint
Palpitations.

History of presenting complaint
Six-month history of intermittent palpitations, feeling like 'missed beats', particularly at rest. Otherwise asymptomatic. No chest pain, breathlessness, pre-syncope or syncope. No prolonged episodes of palpitation.

Past medical history
Nil.

Examination
Pulse: 60/min, occasional irregularity.
Blood pressure: 132/80.
JVP: not elevated.
Heart sounds: normal.
Chest auscultation: unremarkable.
No peripheral oedema.

Investigations
FBC: Hb 14.7, WCC 6.3, platelets 365.
U&E: Na 141, K 4.5, urea 4.8, creatinine 89.
Thyroid function: normal.
Chest X-ray: normal heart size, clear lung fields.

QUESTIONS

1. What rhythm is seen on this ECG?
2. What investigations might be appropriate?
3. What treatment options are available?

ECG ANALYSIS

Rate	60/min
Rhythm	Sinus rhythm with a single ventricular ectopic beat
QRS axis	Normal (+6°)
P waves	Present
PR interval	Normal (140 ms)
QRS duration	Normal (80 ms)
T waves	Normal
QTc interval	Normal (380 ms)

ANSWERS

1. This ECG shows sinus rhythm with a single **ventricular ectopic beat** (VEB).
2. VEBs are often benign, but some patients may be at risk of dangerous ventricular arrhythmias. Assessment should include a full history and examination, and needs to be particularly thorough in those with structural heart disease or risk factors for sudden cardiac death (e.g. family history). Investigations may need to include a check of serum electrolytes, 12-lead ECG, echocardiography, ambulatory ECG monitoring (to quantify the frequency of VEBs and to screen for ventricular tachycardia) and imaging investigations to look for evidence of coronary artery disease.
3. Identify and address any underlying causes (e.g. high caffeine intake, electrolyte abnormalities, myocardial ischaemia, cardiomyopathy). Benign VEBs may require just reassurance, although beta blockers may help if symptoms are troublesome. Patients at risk of dangerous arrhythmias may require catheter ablation or an implantable cardioverter defibrillator.

COMMENTARY

- VEBs, also known as ventricular extrasystoles, ventricular premature complexes (VPCs), ventricular premature beats (VPBs) or premature ventricular contractions (PVCs), are a common finding and are often asymptomatic. They can, however, cause troublesome palpitations and sometimes herald a risk of dangerous arrhythmias. Patients with VEBs therefore require appropriate clinical assessment.
- VEBs cause broad QRS complexes and occur earlier than the next normal beat would have occurred. VEBs may be followed by inverted P waves if the atria are activated by retrograde conduction. If retrograde conduction does not occur, there will usually be a full compensatory pause before the next normal beat because the sinoatrial node will not be 'reset'.
- Two consecutive VEBs are termed a couplet; three or more are termed ventricular tachycardia (VT).
- Multiple VEBs which share the same QRS complex morphology originate from a single focus within the ventricles and are therefore called unifocal. Where VEBs have two or more different morphologies, they arise from different foci and are called multifocal.
- Causes of VEBs include myocardial ischaemia/infarction, electrolyte disturbance (e.g. hypokalaemia, hypomagnesaemia), myocarditis, cardiomyopathy, caffeine, alcohol, sympathomimetic drugs and digoxin toxicity.
- If VEBs are infrequent, and if structural heart disease and documented VT are absent, the prognosis is generally good.
- Beta blockers can be useful in those with troublesome symptoms but otherwise benign VEBs, although reassurance alone may suffice in this patient group. Where feasible, catheter ablation can be considered where symptoms are troublesome or there is a risk of malignant arrhythmias. An implantable cardioverter defibrillator is also an option to provide protection from dangerous arrhythmias.

Further reading

Making Sense of the ECG 4th edition: Ventricular ectopic beats, p 79.

Ng GA. Treating patients with ventricular ectopic beats. *Heart* 2006; **92**: 1707–12.

CASE 10

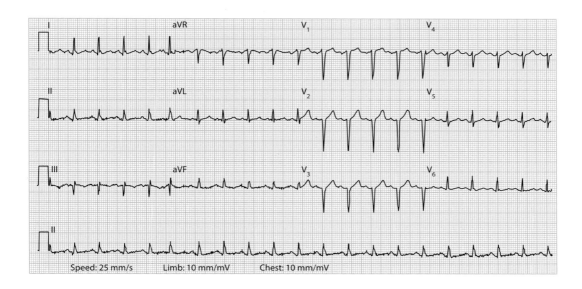

Speed: 25 mm/s   Limb: 10 mm/mV   Chest: 10 mm/mV

CLINICAL SCENARIO

Female, aged 18 years.

Presenting complaint
Palpitations.

History of presenting complaint
Direct questioning reveals that the patient is aware of an episodic fast heart beat, particularly at times of stress and anxiety. Recently started studying at a local college and has been finding the coursework stressful.

Past medical history
Nil of note.

Examination
Pulse: 120/min.
Blood pressure: 118/76.
JVP: not elevated.
Heart sounds: normal.
Chest auscultation: unremarkable.
No peripheral oedema.

Investigations
FBC: Hb 12.9, WCC 6.5, platelets 356.
U&E: Na 141, K 4.1, urea 3.8, creatinine 86.
Thyroid function: normal.
Chest X-ray: normal heart size, clear lung fields.
Echocardiogram: normal valves and normal left ventricular function (ejection fraction 67 per cent).

QUESTIONS

1. What does this ECG show?
2. What are the likely causes?
3. What are the key issues in managing this patient?

ECG ANALYSIS

Rate	120/min
Rhythm	Sinus tachycardia
QRS axis	Normal (+35°)
P waves	Normal
PR interval	Normal (136 ms)
QRS duration	Normal (98 ms)
T waves	Normal
QTc interval	Normal (440 ms)

ANSWERS

1. There is a normally shaped P wave before every QRS complex. This is **sinus tachycardia** (sinus rhythm with a heart rate greater than 100/min).

2. Sinus tachycardia is usually a normal physiological response to physical or emotional stress. There are numerous potential causes, including pain, anaemia, fever, drugs (e.g. adrenaline, atropine, salbutamol (do not forget inhalers and nebulizers), caffeine and alcohol), ischaemic heart disease and acute myocardial infarction, heart failure, pulmonary embolism, fluid loss and hyperthyroidism. Rarely, it can be the result of a primary sinoatrial node abnormality.

3. First, it is important to establish that a tachycardia is indeed sinus tachycardia, as atrial tachycardia and atrial flutter can both resemble sinus tachycardia if the ECG is not inspected carefully enough. Second, a careful assessment of the patient is required to establish the cause of the sinus tachycardia and whether or not it is haemodynamically 'appropriate' (compensating for low blood pressure such as fluid loss or anaemia) or 'inappropriate' (e.g. anxiety, thyrotoxicosis). Third, although beta blockers are effective at slowing sinus tachycardia, using a beta blocker to slow an 'appropriate' sinus tachycardia can lead to haemodynamic decompensation.

COMMENTARY

- Clinical examination is essential. Request thyroid function tests. Catecholamine levels may be abnormal (phaeochromocytoma) – check especially if there is a history of hypertension.
- 'Palpitations' can be documented using:
  - 12-lead ECG – most useful if the patient complains of palpitations during the recording.
  - 24-h (or longer) ambulatory ECG recording – if palpitations are infrequent, the patient will have nothing to record.
  - Cardiomemo – this patient-activated device may be carried for several weeks until an episode of palpitations occurs.
  - Implantable ECG loop recorder – this is particularly useful if palpitations are infrequent but a serious arrhythmia is still suspected. The device is implanted subcutaneously and records the ECG continuously, storing periods that show arrhythmias or coincide with symptoms.
- Symptoms sometimes give a clue as to the underlying rhythm disturbance:
  - Heart 'jumping' or 'missing a beat'– ectopics (atrial or ventricular).
  - Intermittent rapid erratic heartbeat – paroxysmal atrial fibrillation.
  - Sustained rapid regular palpitations with abrupt onset and termination – atrioventricular re-entry tachycardia or atrioventricular nodal re-entry tachycardia.

Further reading

Making Sense of the ECG 4th edition: Sinus tachycardia, p 55; Ambulatory ECG recording, p 217.

Morillo CA, Kleinm GJ, Thakur RK *et al.* Mechanism of 'inappropriate' sinus tachycardia. Role of sympathovagal balance. *Circulation* 1994; **90**: 873–7.

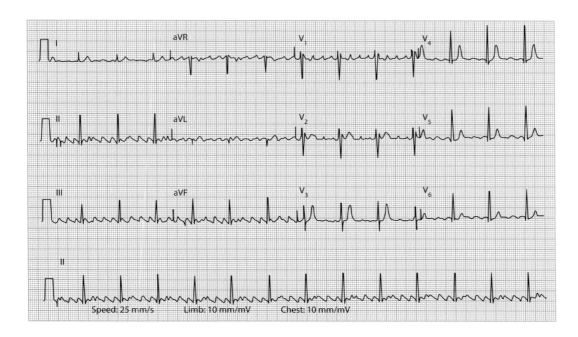

CLINICAL SCENARIO

Male, aged 66 years.

Presenting complaint
Progressive exertional breathlessness.

History of presenting complaint
Normally active, he had noticed a gradual fall in his exercise capacity over a 2-week period prior to presentation. The main limiting factor in his exercise was breathlessness. He had not experienced any orthopnoea or paroxysmal nocturnal dyspnoea, and did not have any peripheral oedema.

Past medical history
Mitral valve prolapse with moderate mitral regurgitation.

Examination
Pulse: 75/min, regular.
Blood pressure: 118/78.
JVP: not elevated.
Heart sounds: 3/6 pansystolic murmur at apex, radiating to axilla.
Chest auscultation: bilateral inspiratory crackles at both lung bases.
No peripheral oedema.

Investigations
FBC: Hb 13.9, WCC 8.1, platelets 233.
U&E: Na 137, K 4.2, urea 5.3, creatinine 88.
Thyroid function: normal.
Troponin I: negative.
Chest X-ray: mild cardiomegaly, early pulmonary congestion.
Echocardiogram: Anterior mitral valve leaflet prolapse with posteriorly directed jet of moderate mitral regurgitation into a moderately dilated left atrium. Left ventricular function mildly impaired (ejection fraction 47 per cent).

QUESTIONS

1. What rhythm does this ECG show?
2. What is the mechanism of this arrhythmia?
3. How can the atrial rhythm be demonstrated more clearly?
4. What are the key issues in managing this arrhythmia?

ECG ANALYSIS

Rate	75/min
Rhythm	Atrial flutter
QRS axis	Normal (+68°)
P waves	Absent – atrial flutter waves are present
PR interval	Not applicable
QRS duration	Normal (80 ms)
T waves	Normal
QTc interval	Normal (358 ms)

Additional comments

The 'sawtooth' pattern of atrial flutter is clearly evident, particularly in the inferior leads (II, III and aVF) and in chest lead V1. There is one QRS complex for every 4 flutter waves (note that one flutter wave is masked by each QRS complex), indicating 4:1 atrioventricular block.

ANSWERS

1. Atrial flutter with 4:1 atrioventricular block.
2. Atrial flutter usually results from a macro re-entry circuit within the right atrium (although other variants are recognized). The atria typically depolarize 300 times/min, giving rise to 300 flutter waves/min. However, depending on the type of atrial flutter, flutter rates can vary between 250/min and 350/min.
3. Flutter waves are best seen in the inferior leads and in lead V1. They can be difficult to see when the ventricular rate is higher (e.g. with 2:1 or 3:1 block) as the flutter waves are masked by the overlying QRS complexes. Temporary blocking of the atrioventricular node with carotid sinus massage or adenosine (except where contraindicated) can block the QRS complexes for a few seconds, revealing the atrial activity more clearly.
4. There are four key aspects to the treatment of atrial flutter:
   - Ventricular rate control – the drugs used for ventricular rate control are the same as those for atrial fibrillation (beta blockers or rate-limiting calcium channel blockers (e.g. verapamil, diltiazem), and/or digoxin).
   - There is a thromboembolic risk, and so consider the patient for antithrombotic therapy in the same way as for atrial fibrillation.
   - Electrical cardioversion can be very effective in restoring sinus rhythm and, as a general rule, atrial flutter is easier to cardiovert than atrial fibrillation.
   - Electrophysiological intervention with radio-frequency ablation of the atrial flutter re-entry circuit is an effective procedure with a success rate >95 per cent.

COMMENTARY

- Atrial flutter is a common arrhythmia. It can occur in association with underlying cardiac disease such as ischaemic heart disease, valvular heart disease and cardiomyopathies, as well as in pulmonary diseases such as pulmonary embolism and chronic obstructive pulmonary disease.
- Although the atria depolarize around 300 times/min in atrial flutter, the atrioventricular node (fortunately) cannot conduct impulses to the ventricles that quickly, so after conducting an impulse the node will remain refractory for the next one, two or even more impulses until it is ready to conduct again. In this example, the node is conducting every fourth flutter wave to the ventricles, giving rise to 4:1 atrioventricular block.
- The heart rate will vary according to the degree of atrioventricular block – ventricular rates often run at 150/min (2:1 block), 100/min (3:1 block) or 75/min (4:1 block). The block can be variable, with a varying heart rate and an irregular pulse.
- Atrial flutter with 2:1 block is particularly common. In cases of 2:1 block the ventricular rate is

around 150/min. Always consider a diagnosis of atrial flutter whenever someone presents with a regular narrow complex tachycardia and a ventricular rate of 150/min.

- The differential diagnosis of atrial flutter includes:
  - Atrial tachycardia – The atrial rate is usually lower and the atrial activity is marked by abnormally shaped P waves rather than flutter waves.
  - Atrial fibrillation – Can be mistaken for atrial flutter with variable block. Atrial activity in atrial fibrillation is less well defined on the ECG than the sawtooth pattern seen in atrial flutter.

Further reading

Making Sense of the ECG 4th edition: Atrial flutter, p 64.

Waldo AL. Treatment of atrial flutter. *Heart* 2000; **84**: 227–32.

CASE 12

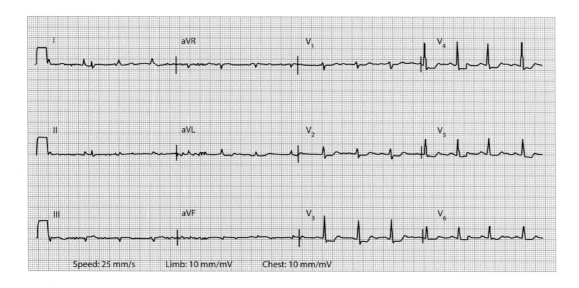

Speed: 25 mm/s   Limb: 10 mm/mV   Chest: 10 mm/mV

CLINICAL SCENARIO

Male, aged 64 years.

Presenting complaint
Severe 'crushing' central chest pain.

History of presenting complaint
Chest pain on exertion for 3 months but put it down to indigestion. Tried over-the-counter antacids and pain eventually got better. However, he was then woken from sleep with severe chest pain. Started to have difficulty breathing.

Past medical history
Hypertension for 10 years.
Smoker of 30 cigarettes per day for 40 years.

Examination
Pulse: 90/min, regular.
Blood pressure: 156/104.
JVP: not elevated.
Heart sounds: normal.
Chest auscultation: unremarkable.
No peripheral oedema.

Investigations
FBC: Hb 15.5, WCC 6.9, platelets 198.
U&E: Na 139, K 5.1, urea 4.4, creatinine 96.
Thyroid function: normal.
Troponin I: normal (at 6 h).
Chest X-ray: no cardiomegaly, mild pulmonary congestion.
Echocardiogram: normal valves. Mild concentric left ventricular hypertrophy. Left ventricular function mildly impaired (ejection fraction 46 per cent).

QUESTIONS

1. What does this ECG show?
2. What is the mechanism of this?
3. What are the key issues in managing this patient?

ECG ANALYSIS

Rate	90/min
Rhythm	Sinus rhythm
QRS axis	Normal (+14°)
P waves	Normal
PR interval	Normal (160 ms)
QRS duration	Normal (90 ms)
T waves	Normal
QTc interval	Normal (440 ms)

Additional comments

There is ST segment depression in leads V2–V6 and aVL.

ANSWERS

1. The ECG shows sinus rhythm. There is ST segment depression in leads V2–V6 and aVL, indicating myocardial ischaemia in the territory of the left anterior descending coronary artery. As the troponin level remained normal at 6 h, this represents unstable angina.
2. The mechanism of this ischaemia is likely to be a reduction in blood flow to the myocardium because of a degree of obstruction to flow down the left anterior descending coronary artery. In view of the clinical presentation (acute coronary syndrome), it is likely that a previously stable coronary endothelial plaque has ruptured, exposing the lipid-rich core. Platelets adhere, change shape and secrete adenosine diphosphate (ADP) and other pro-aggregants; this may 'seal' and stabilize the plaque, but the lumen may be at least partially obstructed, reducing blood flow.
3. Admit the patient to a monitored area. Give pain relief with opiates with or without intravenous nitrates; beta blockers with or without calcium channel blockers; subcutaneous heparin; and anti-platelet treatment with aspirin and clopidogrel. Consider the use of an intravenous glycoprotein IIb/IIIa antagonist (e.g. tirofiban) to 'pacify' the culprit lesion. Check a troponin level to aid diagnosis and help formulate management. Arrange coronary angiography to define coronary anatomy and, as appropriate, to plan coronary revascularization with percutaneous coronary intervention (PCI) or coronary artery bypass grafting.

COMMENTARY

- Cardiac-sounding chest pain may be due to an acute coronary syndrome, classified on the basis of the ECG as:
  - **ST segment elevation myocardial infarction** (STEMI): the ECG shows ST segment elevation and the primary aim of treatment is reopening of the coronary artery and reperfusion of the myocardium, via urgent primary PCI (or thrombolysis depending on local availability).
  - **Non-ST segment elevation acute coronary syndrome** (NSTEACS): the ECG may be normal, or may show ST segment depression or T wave inversion. The primary aim of treatment is urgent antiplatelet, antithrombotic and anti-ischaemic drug treatment, followed by coronary angiography and revascularization as appropriate.
- In the case of NSTEACS, cases are subsequently divided into **non-ST segment elevation myocardial infarction** (NSTEMI) or **unstable angina** (UA) once the troponin (I or T) results become available. The subgroup of patients with an elevated troponin level is classified as having had a NSTEMI; those whose troponin level remains normal are classified as having UA.
- As well as providing a diagnostic label, troponin results are helpful in allowing risk stratification – the degree of troponin elevation predicts a higher risk of future cardiovascular events.

Further reading

Making Sense of the ECG 4th edition: Are the ST segments depressed? p 171; Acute coronary syndromes, p 160.
NICE guideline on unstable angina and NSTEMI (2010) – downloadable from: http://guidance.nice.org.uk/CG94.
Wagner GS, Macfarlane P, Wellens H *et al.* AHA/ACCF/HRS recommendations for the standardization and interpretation of the electrocardiogram: Part VI: Acute ischaemia/infarction. *J Am Coll Cardiol* 2009; **53**: 1003–11.

CASE 13

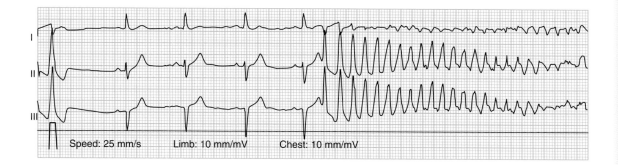

I

II

III

Speed: 25 mm/s   Limb: 10 mm/mV   Chest: 10 mm/mV

CLINICAL SCENARIO

Male, aged 63 years.

Presenting complaint
Six-month history of worsening exertional chest pain.

History of presenting complaint
Listed for urgent coronary angiography to investigate his chest pain. This ECG was recorded during his coronary angiogram, which had revealed a severe left main stem coronary stenosis. The ECG shown above was recorded just after the first injection of contrast into the left coronary artery. The patient complained of chest pain, and then became unresponsive.

Past medical history
Angina.
Type 2 diabetes mellitus.
Hypertension.

Examination
Patient supine in cardiac catheter department, undergoing coronary angiography. Appears pale and clammy.
Blood pressure: 158/88, falling rapidly to become unrecordable while this ECG was recorded. Patient became unresponsive during this ECG recording.

Investigations
FBC: Hb 14.1, WCC 7.6, platelets 304.
U&E: Na 139, K 4.4, urea 6.5, creatinine 84.
Glucose: 8.3 (known diabetes).

QUESTIONS

1. What does this ECG show?
2. What immediate action should be taken?
3. What medium-term action should be taken?

ECG ANALYSIS

Rate	52/min (during sinus rhythm), then unmeasurable
Rhythm	Sinus rhythm with ventricular ectopics, followed by ventricular tachycardia (VT) which rapidly degenerates into ventricular fibrillation (VF)
QRS axis	Left axis deviation (the axis moves increasingly leftward during the four sinus beats)
P waves	Present for the sinus beats, then absent during VT/VF
PR interval	Normal during sinus beats (160 ms)
QRS duration	Normal during sinus beats (110 ms)
T waves	Normal during sinus beats
QTc interval	Normal during sinus beats (392 ms)

Additional comments

The ventricular tachycardia (VT) is triggered by a ventricular ectopic beat (VEB) occurring during the T wave of the fourth sinus beat (R on T ectopic).

ANSWERS

1. The ECG shows a ventricular ectopic, followed by four normal sinus beats. Another VEB then occurs during the T wave of the fourth sinus beat (R on T ectopic), triggering pulseless VT which then rapidly degenerates into VF.
2. The patient has sustained a cardiac arrest (pulseless VT/VF). As this was a witnessed and monitored arrest, a precordial thump can be given followed, if unsuccessful, by defibrillation. In this case, the patient did not respond to a precordial thump but sinus rhythm was restored following a single biphasic shock of 150 J. The patient should then be reassessed with regards to their airway, breathing and circulation.
3. Following successful resuscitation, transfer the patient to a coronary or intensive care unit for monitoring of airway and breathing (including pulse oximetry), vital signs (pulse, blood pressure (preferably via an arterial line) and temperature), peripheral perfusion, cardiac rhythm, neurological status (including Glasgow Coma Score) and urine output and fluid balance. In addition, check arterial blood gases, blood urea and electrolytes (including potassium, magnesium and calcium), chest X-ray and blood glucose, 12-lead ECG and full blood count. In view of the critical nature of the patient's coronary disease, arrange urgent revascularization.

COMMENTARY

- VF is characterized by its chaotic waveform with no discernible organized ventricular activity, in the context of a patient who is pulseless. A precordial thump is seldom successful in restoring sinus rhythm, but it is worth a single attempt at a precordial thump if the arrest was witnessed and monitored, and DC cardioversion is not immediately available. Lose no time, however, in obtaining a defibrillator and administering a shock.
- VEBs that fall on the T wave (R on T ventricular ectopics) occur during ventricular repolarization, which is a vulnerable time for ventricular arrhythmias. As the ventricles repolarize, they do so in a 'patchy' fashion, meaning that some areas of the myocardium repolarize more quickly than others. This leads to islands of refractory myocardium, surrounded by myocardium that has repolarized. A ventricular ectopic arising at this time can establish a re-entry circuit around one of these refractory islands, causing VT which can then degenerate into VF.
- The VEBs and consequent pulseless VT/VF were, in this case, related to the patient's critical coronary disease. The left main stem is a critically important part of the coronary arteries and ischaemia or infarction arising from a left main stem stenosis will affect a large proportion of the left ventricle.
- Although arrhythmias account for 35 per cent of all complications during coronary angiography, they account for only 12 per cent of deaths, reflecting the careful monitoring of patients in the cardiac catheter department and the high level of expertise of staff in advanced life support.

Further reading

Making Sense of the ECG 4th edition: Ventricular fibrillation, p 90; Ventricular ectopic beats, p 79.

Resuscitation Council (UK). Resuscitation guidelines. 2010. Available at: www.resus.org.uk.

CASE 14

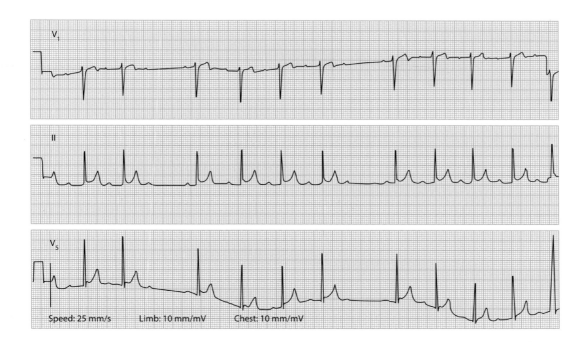

V₁

II

V₅

Speed: 25 mm/s   Limb: 10 mm/mV   Chest: 10 mm/mV

CLINICAL SCENARIO

Male, aged 66 years.

Presenting complaint
Sensation of 'missed heartbeats'.

History of presenting complaint
After retiring, and adopting a more sedentary lifestyle, the patient first became aware of something wrong when he was sitting quietly, reading the newspaper. He noticed that every now and then, his heart appeared to 'miss a beat'. Although he still enjoyed his normal weekend walking and badminton, he was anxious in case the missed beats were a sign of heart disease, as his mother had recently died of a 'massive heart attack'. He reported his concerns to his family doctor.

Past medical history
No significant medical history.

Examination
Pulse: 57/min, irregular (occasional 'missed beats').
Blood pressure: 144/94.
JVP: not elevated.
Heart sounds: normal.
Chest auscultation: unremarkable.
No peripheral oedema.

Investigations
FBC: Hb 14.3, WCC 7.5, platelets 278.
U&E: Na 139, K 5.0, urea 5.1, creatinine 96.
Chest X-ray: normal heart size, clear lung fields.
Echocardiogram: normal.

QUESTIONS

1. What does this ECG show?
2. What is the mechanism of this?
3. What is the prognosis?
4. How should this be managed?

ECG ANALYSIS

Rate	57/min
Rhythm	Sinus rhythm with second-degree atrioventricular block (Mobitz type I)
QRS axis	Unable to assess (rhythm strip)
P waves	Normal
PR interval	Variable – gradually lengthens before 'resetting' after a nonconducted P wave
QRS duration	Normal (110 ms)
T waves	Normal
QTc interval	Normal (400 ms)

ANSWERS

1. The PR interval gradually increases after each successive P wave until one P wave is not conducted at all, resulting in a 'missed beat'. After this, conduction reverts to normal and the cycle starts over again. This is an example of second-degree atrioventricular block of the Mobitz type I (Wenckebach phenomenon) subtype.

2. One can imagine Mobitz type I atrioventricular block as the atrioventricular node becoming increasingly 'tired' as it conducts each P wave – as a result, the node takes longer and longer to conduct each subsequent P wave until it totally 'gives up' and fails to conduct a P wave at all. This however gives the atrioventricular node a chance to 'rest', and by the time the next P wave arrives it is ready to conduct normally, before the cycle repeats itself.

3. Mobitz type I atrioventricular block occurring at the level of the atrioventricular node has often been described as 'benign' (although pacing is indicated if symptomatic). However, there is disagreement between European and US cardiologists over prognosis – European guidelines support pacing for *asymptomatic* Mobitz type I atrioventricular block, because of concerns over the risk of progression to higher degrees of atrioventricular block. US guidelines do not support this approach.

4. Chronic *symptomatic* Mobitz type I atrioventricular block should be paced (class I indication).

There is however a disagreement between European and US guidelines on *asymptomatic* Mobitz type I atrioventricular block. European guidelines support pacing for acquired asymptomatic Mobitz type I atrioventricular block as a class IIa indication. However, American guidelines advise against permanent pacemaker implantation for asymptomatic Mobitz type I atrioventricular block at the AV node level (or which is not known to be intra- or infra-Hisian) (class III indication). When the block is infranodal (as identified by electrophysiological testing) there is a stronger indication for pacing.

COMMENTARY

- 'Palpitations' can be difficult to document, especially if they are infrequent, of short duration or associated with sudden collapse. Options are:
  - Prolonged (or repeated) Holter recording for 24, 48 or 72 h duration – this will record every heart beat for a set period and will help determine whether the patient's perceived 'palpitation' is related to a cardiac problem. It is especially useful when symptoms occur on most days.
  - If there are no events to record, the patient may be given a patient-activated Cardiomemo device – this can be carried for much longer periods (weeks if necessary) until the patient reports that a 'palpitation' has occurred.

- In a few patients, symptoms may still be suspected to be due to a cardiac arrhythmia but are not frequent enough for short ambulatory recordings to be practical. An implantable ECG loop recorder may help. About the size and shape of a small computer 'memory stick', a loop recorder is implanted under local anaesthesia, just below the skin of the left chest wall. Although the device records continuously, the patient is taught how to electronically document when an event occurred so that the timing of the event can be checked against the cardiac rhythm at that time. The device can also automatically store rhythm strips when it detects a suspected rhythm disturbance.

Further reading

Making Sense of the ECG 4th edition: Second degree atrioventricular block, p 94; Mobitz type I atrioventricular block, p 95; Indications for permanent pacing, p 211.

Sutton R. Mobitz type 1 second degree atrioventricular block: the value of permanent pacing in the older patient. *Heart* 2013; **99**: 291–2.

CASE 15

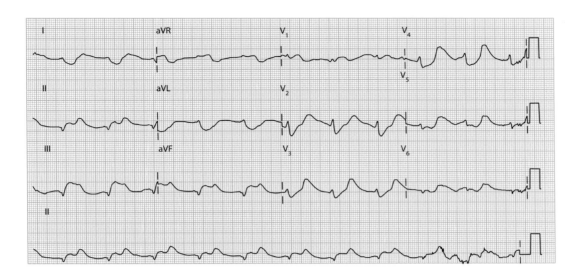

CLINICAL SCENARIO

Female, aged 77 years.

Presenting complaint
Fatigue and feeling generally unwell.

History of presenting complaint
Known chronic renal impairment. One-week history of diarrhoea and vomiting, with very poor fluid intake. Presented with fatigue and feeling generally unwell.

Past medical history
Chronic renal impairment.

Examination
Patient appears dehydrated and unwell.
Pulse: 66/min, regular.
Blood pressure: 88/44.
JVP: low.
Heart sounds: normal.
Chest auscultation: unremarkable.
No peripheral oedema.
No urine output following urinary catheterization.

Investigations
FBC: Hb 10.8, WCC 22.1, platelets 211.
U&E: Na 130, K 8.2, urea 32.7, creatinine 642.

QUESTIONS

1. What does this ECG show?
2. What is the cause?

ECG ANALYSIS

Rate	66/min
Rhythm	Either sinus rhythm (with undetectable P waves) or junctional rhythm
QRS axis	Unable to assess in view of bizarre QRS complex morphology
P waves	Not visible
PR interval	Not applicable
QRS duration	Broad, bizarre complexes
T waves	Large, broad
QTc interval	Prolonged (>500 ms)

ANSWERS

1. This ECG shows absent P waves and broad, bizarre QRS complexes. With increasing potassium levels, the P waves become smaller in size before disappearing altogether. Patients can also develop sinoatrial and atrioventricular block. The rhythm here may therefore be sinus rhythm with such small P waves that they are no longer evident, or a junctional rhythm (although junctional rhythms are usually slower).

2. The cause of these ECG appearances is severe hyperkalaemia – the patient's potassium level is markedly elevated at 8.2 mmol/L. This has developed as a result of acute-on-chronic renal failure, which is likely to have been precipitated by dehydration.

COMMENTARY

- In general, hyperkalaemia causes a sequence of ECG changes at different potassium levels:
  - early ECG changes include tall 'tented' T waves, shortening of the QT interval and ST segment depression
  - at higher potassium levels, the QRS complexes become broad and there is lengthening of the PR interval (with flattening or even loss of the P wave)
  - sinoatrial and atrioventricular block can develop
  - at very high potassium levels, the QRS complexes become increasingly bizarre and merge with the T waves to resemble a sine wave
  - arrhythmias (including ventricular fibrillation and asystole) can occur at any point.
- There is considerable variation in the ECG appearances between individuals with hyperkalaemia. Some patients will develop quite marked ECG abnormalities with fairly modest hyperkalaemia, while others can have minor ECG changes despite severe hyperkalaemia.
- Because of the risk of life-threatening arrhythmias, patients with hyperkalaemia need continuous ECG monitoring.
- If the diagnosis of hyperkalaemia is confirmed by an elevated plasma potassium level, assess the patient for symptoms and signs of an underlying cause (e.g. renal failure, as in this case). In particular, review their treatment chart for inappropriate potassium supplements and potassium-sparing diuretics.
- Hyperkalaemia needs urgent treatment if it is causing ECG abnormalities or the plasma potassium level is above 6.5 mmol/L.

Further reading

Making Sense of the ECG 4th edition: Hyperkalaemia, p 180.

Montague BT, Ouellette JR, Buller GK. Retrospective review of the frequency of ECG changes in hyperkalemia. *Clin J Am Soc Nephrol* 2008; **3**: 324–30.

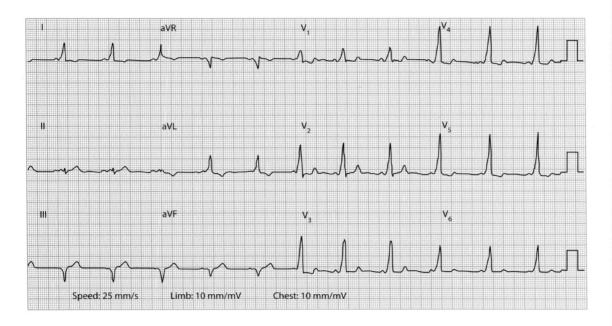

Speed: 25 mm/s   Limb: 10 mm/mV   Chest: 10 mm/mV

CLINICAL SCENARIO

Male, aged 26 years.

Presenting complaint
Asymptomatic.

History of presenting complaint
Incidental finding when attending for private insurance medical.

Past medical history
Nil of note.

Examination
Pulse: 66/min, regular.
Blood pressure: 126/84.
JVP: normal.
Heart sounds: normal.
Chest auscultation: unremarkable.
No peripheral oedema.

Investigations
FBC: Hb 16.2, WCC 6.4, platelets 332.
U&E: Na 141, K 4.9, urea 5.5, creatinine 90.
Chest X-ray: normal heart size, clear lung fields.
Echocardiogram: normal.

QUESTIONS

1. What does this ECG show?
2. What is the mechanism of this?
3. What are the possible causes?
4. What are the key issues in managing this patient?

ECG ANALYSIS

Rate	66/min
Rhythm	Sinus rhythm
QRS axis	Normal (−24°)
P waves	Normal
PR interval	Short (90 ms)
QRS duration	Lengthened (160 ms)
T waves	Normal
QTc interval	Normal (452 ms)

Additional comments

A delta wave is present (an initial slurred upstroke on the QRS complexes).

ANSWERS

1. A P wave precedes every QRS complex so the rhythm is sinus rhythm. However, the PR interval is short, and there is slurring of the initial part of the QRS complex producing a delta wave, clearly visible in leads I, aVL and V1–V6. This is the **Wolff–Parkinson–White (WPW) ECG pattern.**

2. Conduction from atria to ventricles is usually through a single connection involving the atrioventricular (AV) node and bundle of His. In patients with WPW ECG pattern, a second or 'accessory' pathway (the bundle of Kent) coexists, and conducts an electrical signal from the atria to the ventricles at a faster rate than through the AV node, which means that the PR interval is shorter than normal. As a result, the ventricles are activated by the accessory pathway before the impulse has (simultaneously) been transmitted through the AV node – known as ventricular pre-excitation. It causes the delta-shaped upstroke of the R wave. Eventually the impulse via the AV node catches up and fuses with the impulse depolarizing the ventricles via the accessory pathway, so that the remainder of ventricular depolarization occurs normally.

3. During fetal development, the atria and ventricles are separated electrically, with a single connection through the AV node and bundle of His. This protects the ventricles from rapid atrial activity, as the refractory period of the AV node places an upper limit on how rapidly atrial impulses can be transmitted to the ventricles. Incomplete separation leaves an accessory pathway, most often located in the left free wall or postero-septal wall, bypassing the AV node. Occasionally multiple pathways exist.

4. Patients may remain asymptomatic. Some patients with a WPW ECG pattern experience episodes of atrioventricular re-entry tachycardia (AVRT), in which case they are said to have **WPW syndrome.** This can be treated pharmacologically or with ablation of the accessory pathway.

COMMENTARY

- Symptoms of AVRT are very variable. Patients complain of 'palpitations', usually of sudden onset and abrupt termination. The palpitations vary greatly in duration and severity, and may be accompanied by chest pain, dizziness or syncope.

- With anterograde conduction via the AV node and retrograde conduction via the accessory pathway, an orthodromic AVRT is said to occur. This is the commoner type of AVRT and during the tachycardia, the delta wave is lost. An AVRT taking the opposite route (down the accessory pathway and up the AV node) is said to be antidromic. This is rarer, and when it does occur, only delta waves are seen as the whole of the ventricular mass is activated via the accessory pathway.

- Some patients do not have any rhythm disturbance and the finding of a WPW ECG pattern is made incidentally when an ECG is recorded for an unrelated problem. Patients who are asymptomatic should nonetheless be seen by a cardiac electrophysiologist to assess their risk of potentially hazardous arrhythmias (e.g. rapidly-conducted atrial fibrillation) in the future.

Further reading

Making Sense of the ECG 4th edition: Wolff–Parkinson–White syndrome, p 69; atrioventricular re-entry tachycardia, p 67.

Keating L, Morris FP, Brady WJ. Electrocardiographic features of Wolff-Parkinson-White syndrome. *Emerg Med J* 2003; **20**: 491–3.

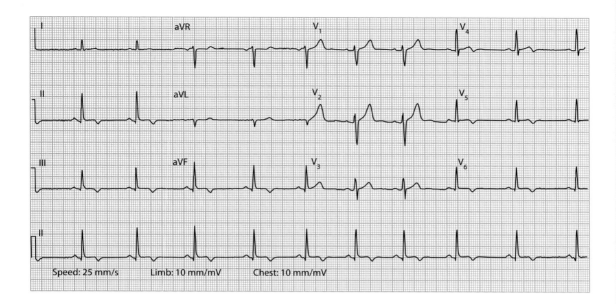

Speed: 25 mm/s   Limb: 10 mm/mV   Chest: 10 mm/mV

CLINICAL SCENARIO

Male, aged 37 years.

Presenting complaint
Severe central chest pain.

History of presenting complaint
Four-hour history of heavy central chest pain, radiating to the left arm and associated with breathlessness and sweating. Chest pain resolved after administration of opiates on arrival in hospital. This ECG was performed 24 h after presentation.

Past medical history
Hypertension diagnosed 2 years ago.
Ex-smoker (15 pack-year smoking history).

Examination
Pulse: 60/min, regular.
Blood pressure: 166/102.
JVP: not elevated.
Heart sounds: normal.
Chest auscultation: unremarkable.
No peripheral oedema.

Investigations
FBC: Hb 15.3, WCC 9.8, platelets 271.
U&E: Na 139, K 4.0, urea 5.8, creatinine 81.
Chest X-ray: normal heart size, clear lung fields.
Troponin I: elevated at 111 (after 6 h).
Echocardiogram: hypokinesia of inferolateral walls of left ventricle, overall ejection fraction 50 per cent.

QUESTIONS

1. What abnormalities does this ECG show?
2. What is the diagnosis?
3. What treatment is indicated?

ECG ANALYSIS

Rate	60/min
Rhythm	Sinus rhythm
QRS axis	Normal (+73°)
P waves	Normal
PR interval	Normal (140 ms)
QRS duration	Normal (100 ms)
T waves	T wave inversion in leads II, III, aVF, V5–V6 and a biphasic T wave in lead V4
QTc interval	Normal (420 ms)

ANSWERS

1. This ECG shows inferolateral T wave inversion (leads II, III, aVF, V5–V6, with a biphasic T wave in lead V4).

2. The ECG indicates an inferolateral non-ST elevation acute coronary syndrome (NSTEACS). The elevated troponin levels confirm myocardial damage, and therefore a diagnosis **of inferolateral non-ST segment elevation myocardial infarction (NSTEMI)** can be made. In patients in whom the cardiac markers are not elevated 6 h after the onset of chest pain, myocardial infarction can be ruled out, and the diagnosis would be one of unstable angina.

3. The initial treatment of NSTEACS includes:
   - aspirin
   - clopidogrel
   - heparin
   - beta blocker
   - nitrates
   - statin
   - oxygen (if hypoxic) and analgesia as appropriate.
   - glycoprotein IIb/IIIa inhibitor (if indicated).

   Patient requires urgent coronary angiography with a view to coronary revascularization with percutaneous coronary intervention (PCI) or coronary artery bypass grafting as appropriate.

COMMENTARY

- An urgent ECG is required in any patient presenting with cardiac-sounding chest pain. Acute coronary syndromes (ACS) can be divided into ST segment elevation myocardial infarction (STEMI) and non-ST segment elevation ACS (NSTEACS) on the basis of the ECG appearances. The ECG of a patient with NSTEACS may show ST segment depression, T wave inversion or may be normal.

- The differential diagnosis of T wave inversion includes:
  - myocardial ischaemia
  - myocardial infarction
  - ventricular hypertrophy with 'strain'
  - digoxin effect.

- T wave inversion is normal in leads aVR and V1, and in some patients can be a variant of normal in leads V2, V3 and III. An inverted T wave is also normal in lead aVL if it follows a negative QRS complex.

- The location of ischaemic changes on an ECG is an indicator of the myocardial territory affected:

Leads containing ST segment/T wave changes	Location of event
V1–V4	Anterior
I, aVL, V5–V6	Lateral
I, aVL, V1–V6	Anterolateral
V1–V3	Anteroseptal
II, III, aVF	Inferior
I, aVL, V5–V6, II, III, aVF	Inferolateral

- It is important to risk-stratify patients with ACS using a risk estimation tool, such as the TIMI Risk Score (www.timi.org) or the GRACE Registry Risk Score (www.outcomes-umassmed.org/grace), as this will help to guide the management strategy.

Further reading

Making Sense of the ECG 4th edition: Are any of the T waves inverted? p 183.

Peters RJG, Mehta S, Yusuf S. Acute coronary syndromes without ST segment elevation. *BMJ* 2007; **334**: 1265–9.

CASE 18

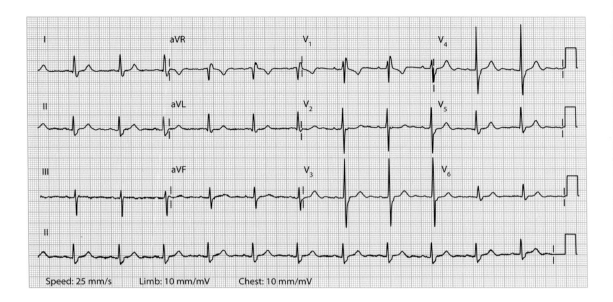

Speed: 25 mm/s   Limb: 10 mm/mV   Chest: 10 mm/mV

CLINICAL SCENARIO

Male, aged 44 years.

Presenting complaint
Awaiting minor surgery. Attended hospital for preoperative assessment.

History of presenting complaint
Asymptomatic; incidental finding.

Past medical history
Fit and well – keen tennis player.
No significant medical history.

Examination
Pulse: 66/min, regular.
Blood pressure: 134/90.
JVP: normal.
Heart sounds: normal.
Chest auscultation: unremarkable.
No peripheral oedema.

Investigations
FBC: Hb 16.1, WCC 5.7, platelets 320.
U&E: Na 140, K 4.7, urea 4.5, creatinine 94.
Chest X-ray: normal heart size, clear lung fields.
Echocardiogram: normal.

QUESTIONS

1. What does this ECG show?
2. What is the mechanism of this?
3. What are the likely causes?
4. What are the key issues in managing this patient?

ECG ANALYSIS

Rate	66/min
Rhythm	Sinus rhythm
QRS axis	Normal (−11°)
P waves	Normal
PR interval	Normal (180 ms)
QRS duration	Prolonged (140 ms)
T waves	Normal
QTc interval	Mildly prolonged (460 ms)

Additional comments

The QRS complexes have a right bundle branch block morphology.

ANSWERS

1. The QRS complexes are broad (140 ms) and the QRS complex in lead V1 has a rSR′ ('M' shape) morphology. This is **right bundle branch block (RBBB)**.
2. In RBBB the interventricular septum depolarizes normally from left to right. The electrical impulse then passes down the left bundle so the left ventricle depolarizes normally, but depolarization of the right ventricle is delayed because the depolarization has to occur via the left ventricle, travelling from myocyte to myocyte, rather than directly via the Purkinje fibres. This leads to a broad QRS complex with the characteristic rSR′ morphology in lead V1.
3. RBBB is a relatively common finding in normal hearts, but can be a marker of underlying disease including ischaemic heart disease, cardiomyopathy, atrial septal defect, Ebstein's anomaly, Fallot's tetralogy and pulmonary embolism (usually massive). It can also occur at fast heart rates in supraventricular tachycardia – this may lead to an incorrect diagnosis of ventricular tachycardia. Incomplete RBBB is found in 2–3 per cent of normal individuals and is usually of no clinical significance.
4. RBBB does not cause symptoms and does not require treatment. However, it is a prompt to look for an underlying cause. Investigations should be appropriate for the clinical presentation.

COMMENTARY

- RBBB may be intermittent, occurring during episodes of tachycardia (when the heart rate exceeds the refractory period of the right bundle). Although both right and left bundle branch block can be 'rate-related' in this way, the right bundle is more likely to be affected.
- An RBBB morphology is seen in Brugada syndrome, in association with persistent ST segment elevation in leads V1–V3. Brugada syndrome is an important diagnosis to make as it predisposes individuals to syncope and sudden death due to ventricular arrhythmias (see Case 68). It probably accounts for 50 per cent of sudden cardiac death with an apparently 'normal' heart. Although the ECG has an RBBB morphology in Brugada syndrome, this is not due to RBBB as such but rather is due to abnormal ventricular repolarization.

Further reading

Making Sense of the ECG 4th edition: Bundle branch block, p 153; Right bundle branch block, p 99; Brugada syndrome, p 170.

CASE 19

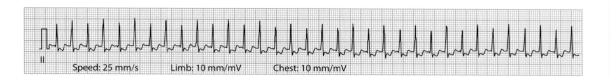

Speed: 25 mm/s   Limb: 10 mm/mV   Chest: 10 mm/mV

CLINICAL SCENARIO

Male, aged 21 years.

Presenting complaint
Rapid regular palpitations.

History of presenting complaint
Normally fit and well with no prior history of palpitations. The patient presented with a 3 h history of rapid regular palpitation.

Past medical history
Wolff–Parkinson–White syndrome diagnosed at age 21 on a routine ECG at an insurance medical.

Examination
Pulse: 204/min, regular.
Blood pressure: 126/80.
JVP: normal.
Heart sounds: normal (tachycardic).
Chest auscultation: unremarkable.

Investigations
FBC: Hb 15.5, WCC 6.2, platelets 347.
U&E: Na 143, K 4.9, urea 4.6, creatinine 68.
Thyroid function: normal.
Chest X-ray: normal heart size, clear lung fields.

QUESTIONS

1. What does this ECG show?
2. What is the underlying pathophysiological mechanism?
3. What initial treatment would be appropriate?
4. What treatment might be appropriate in the longer term?

ECG ANALYSIS

Rate	204/min
Rhythm	Atrioventricular re-entry tachycardia (AVRT)
QRS axis	Unable to assess (single lead)
P waves	Inverted P waves after each QRS complex (distorting the ST segment/T wave)
PR interval	Not applicable
QRS duration	Normal (80 ms)
T waves	Distorted by inverted P waves
QTc interval	Normal (406 ms)

ANSWERS

1. Atrioventricular re-entry tachycardia (AVRT).
2. A re-entry circuit involving an accessory pathway – in this case, the bundle of Kent in Wolff–Parkinson–White (WPW) syndrome. The re-entry circuit travels from atria to ventricles down through the AV node, as per normal, but then travels back up to the atria retrogradely via the accessory pathway. This is known as an orthodromic AVRT (in contrast to an antidromic AVRT, in which the re-entry circuit travels in the opposite direction, down the accessory pathway and back up the AV node).
3. Transiently blocking the AV node can terminate the AVRT. Methods to achieve this include:
   - Valsalva manoeuvre
   - carotid sinus massage
   - intravenous adenosine
   - intravenous verapamil.
4. The patient can be taught the Valsalva manoeuvre to try to terminate episodes. Treatment with maintenance anti-arrhythmic drugs (e.g. sotalol, flecainide, propafenone) can be used to try to prevent recurrent AVRT, but an electrophysiological study with a view to a radiofrequency ablation procedure is often preferable to long-term drug treatment in symptomatic patients.

COMMENTARY

- Patients with a WPW pattern on their ECG have an accessory pathway (the bundle of Kent) that provides an anatomical substrate for the development of AVRT – once an episode of AVRT occurs, the patient is said to have WPW syndrome. Not all patients with a WPW ECG pattern will experience AVRT, however, and some can live out their full life without ever experiencing an episode of AVRT.
- Where WPW patients do get episodes of AVRT, this is usually orthodromic. Orthodromic AVRT is characterized by a narrow-complex tachycardia in which the delta wave is absent during the tachycardia (even though it is present during normal sinus rhythm) and the P waves are seen *after* the QRS complexes, and are inverted in the inferior leads. In the ECG presented here, inverted P waves can be seen at the junction of the ST segment and the T wave.
- AVRT is around 10 times less common than AV *nodal* re-entry tachycardia (AVNRT), which is caused by a micro re-entry circuit within the AV node. P waves are usually easier to discern in AVRT than in AVNRT, and the ECG in sinus rhythm in patients with a history of AVNRT is usually normal, but in those with a history of AVRT it may reveal a short PR interval or delta wave. The distinction between AVRT and AVNRT can be difficult, however, and may require electrophysiological studies.

Further reading

Making Sense of the ECG 4th edition: atrioventricular re-entry tachycardia, p 67; Wolff–Parkinson–White syndrome, p 69.

Whinnett ZI, Sohaib SMA, Davies DW. Diagnosis and management of supraventricular tachycardia. *BMJ* 2012; **345**: e7769.

CASE 20

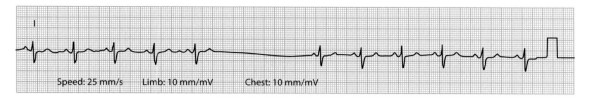

Speed: 25 mm/s   Limb: 10 mm/mV   Chest: 10 mm/mV

CLINICAL SCENARIO

Male, aged 75 years.

Presenting complaint
Syncope.

History of presenting complaint
Brought to emergency department feeling unwell after an episode of collapse with loss of consciousness. Reported several episodes of dizziness in past few months. Quickly back to normal within minutes but episodes tend to reoccur.

Past medical history
Osteoarthritis.

Examination
Pulse: 75/min, regular with occasional 'dropped beat'.
Blood pressure: 156/96.
JVP: normal.
Heart sounds: normal.
Chest auscultation: unremarkable.
No peripheral oedema.

Investigations
FBC: Hb 13.9, WCC 8.1, platelets 233.
U&E: Na 137, K 4.2, urea 5.3, creatinine 88.
Thyroid function: normal.
Troponin I: negative.
Chest X-ray: normal.
Echocardiogram: normal.

QUESTIONS

1. What does this ECG show?
2. What are the likely causes?
3. What are the key issues in managing this patient?

ECG ANALYSIS

Rate	75/min
Rhythm	Sinus rhythm with intermittent sinoatrial block
QRS axis	Unable to assess (rhythm strip)
P waves	Normal (when present)
PR interval	Normal (172 ms)
QRS duration	Normal (98 ms)
T waves	Normal
QTc interval	Normal (440 ms)

ANSWERS

1. The underlying rhythm is normal sinus rhythm but then a P wave fails to appear; the next P wave appears after a pause of 2.4 s. The R-R interval is 0.8 s, so the P wave has arrived 'on schedule', three complete cycle lengths after the last P wave. This is **sinoatrial block**, one of several types of sinus node dysfunction.

2. Sinoatrial node exit block may result from idiopathic fibrosis of the sinus node. Other causes include ischaemic heart disease, myocarditis, cardiomyopathy, cardiac surgery (especially atrial septal defect repair), drugs (such as beta blockers and rate-limiting calcium channel blockers) and digoxin toxicity, excessive vagal tone, and many inflammatory and infiltrative disorders.

3. Asymptomatic sinus node dysfunction does not require treatment, but address any underlying causes (e.g. drugs that can contribute to sinus node dysfunction should be withdrawn). Permanent pacing is appropriate for symptomatic patients (as in this example).

COMMENTARY

- Sinoatrial block should be distinguished from sinus arrest. In sinoatrial block there is a pause with one or more absent P waves, and then the next P wave appears exactly where predicted – in other words, the sinoatrial node continues to 'keep time', but its impulses are not transmitted beyond the node to the atria. In sinus node arrest, the node itself stops firing for a variable time period, so the next P wave occurs after a variable interval.

- Sinoatrial block and sinus arrest can both be features of sick sinus syndrome. Other features of sick sinus syndrome can include sinus bradycardia, brady-tachy syndrome and atrial fibrillation.

- Offer appropriate advice to patients who drive a vehicle and who suffer from presyncope or syncope – very often, they will be barred from driving until the problem has been diagnosed and/or corrected as appropriate. Driving regulations vary between countries. In the UK, information on the medical aspects of fitness to drive can be found on the website of the Driver and Vehicle Licensing Agency (www. dvla.gov.uk).

Further reading

Making Sense of the ECG 4th edition: Sinoatrial block, p 94.

Epstein AE, DiMarco JP, Ellenbogen KA *et al.* ACC/AHA/HRS 2008 Guidelines for device-based therapy of cardiac rhythm abnormalities. *J Am Coll Cardiol* 2008; **51**: e1–62.

The Task Force for Cardiac Pacing and Cardiac Resynchronization Therapy of the European Society of Cardiology (ESC). 2013 ESC guidelines on cardiac pacing and cardiac resynchronization therapy. *Eur Heart J* 2013; **34**: 2281–329.

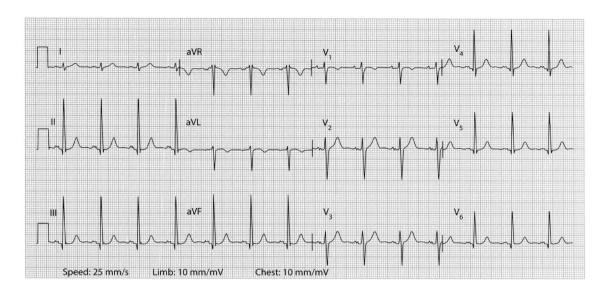

Speed: 25 mm/s   Limb: 10 mm/mV   Chest: 10 mm/mV

CLINICAL SCENARIO

Female, aged 78 years.

Presenting complaint
Exertional breathlessness and fatigue.

History of presenting complaint
One-year history of gradual onset exertional breathlessness and fatigue, with steady fall in exercise capacity.

Past medical history
Rheumatic fever aged 12 years.

Examination
Pulse: 84/min, regular.

Blood pressure: 118/70.
JVP: elevated by 2 cm.
Heart sounds: loud first heart sound (S_1) with an opening snap. Low-pitched 2/6 mid-diastolic murmur with pre-systolic accentuation heard at apex. Loud pulmonary component to second heart sound (P_2).
Chest auscultation: unremarkable.
Mild peripheral oedema.

Investigations
FBC: Hb 12.8, WCC 5.7, platelets 189.
U&E: Na 140, K 4.1, urea 3.7, creatinine 84.
Chest X-ray: large left atrium.

QUESTIONS

1. What does this ECG show?
2. What is the likely cause?
3. What would be the most helpful investigation?
4. What treatment is available?

ECG ANALYSIS

Rate	84/min
Rhythm	Sinus rhythm
QRS axis	Normal (+87°)
P waves	Broad, bifid
PR interval	Normal (150 ms)
QRS duration	Normal (100 ms)
T waves	Normal
QTc interval	Normal (450 ms)

ANSWERS

1. The P waves are broad and bifid ('P mitrale').
2. In the clinical context, the most likely cause is left atrial enlargement secondary to rheumatic mitral stenosis. The clinical features are in keeping with severe mitral stenosis and associated pulmonary hypertension.
3. An echocardiogram would allow direct visualization of the mitral valve, measurement of left atrial size and an estimation of pulmonary artery pressure.
4. Correction of the mitral stenosis is indicated, using percutaneous balloon mitral valvuloplasty, surgical mitral valvotomy or mitral valve replacement.

COMMENTARY

- P mitrale results from enlargement of the left atrium. The enlarged atrium takes longer to depolarize, and thus the P wave becomes broader. Although P mitrale does not require treatment in its own right, its presence should alert you to look for left atrial enlargement. This often results from mitral valve disease, but can also result from left ventricular hypertrophy (the elevated filling pressures of the 'stiff' left ventricle causes gradual enlargement of the left atrium).
- Decisions about which operative intervention to use in mitral stenosis depend primarily on the morphology of the mitral valve and its associated structures. Clear imaging of the valve is therefore essential, and most patients will require a transoesophageal echocardiogram to examine the valve in detail.
- Patients with severe mitral stenosis often develop atrial fibrillation. The consequent loss of P waves means that the ECG evidence of left atrial enlargement is lost.

Further reading

Making Sense of the ECG 4th edition: Are any P waves too wide? p 124.

Prendergast BD, Shaw TRD, Iung B *et al.* Contemporary criteria for the selection of patients for percutaneous balloon mitral valvuloplasty. *Heart* 2002; **87**: 401–4.

CASE 22

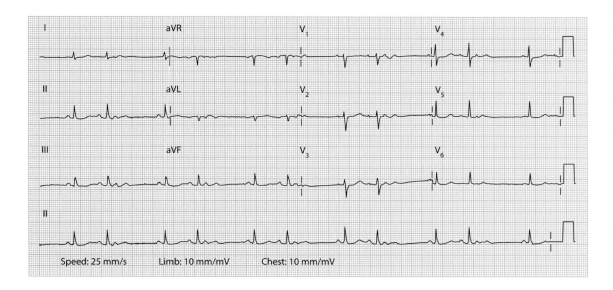

CLINICAL SCENARIO

Male, aged 56 years.

Presenting complaint

Episodes of irregular heart beat; occasionally feeling faint.

History of presenting complaint

For several weeks the patient had been afraid to leave his house due to frequent periods of feeling dizzy. Collapsed on two occasions, waking to find himself on the floor. Back to normal in minutes. Eventually sought advice of a doctor when he collapsed in the toilet and hit his head on the door.

Past medical history

Angina.
Hypertension.

Examination

Pulse: 66/min, regular with frequent 'dropped' beats.
Blood pressure: 156/86.
JVP: not elevated.
Heart sounds: normal.
Chest auscultation: unremarkable.
No peripheral oedema.

Investigations

FBC: Hb 12.2, WCC 8.4, platelets 342.
U&E: Na 137, K 4.2, urea 5.3, creatinine 88.
Thyroid function: normal.
Troponin I: negative.
Chest X-ray: normal heart size, clear lung fields.
Echocardiogram: structurally normal valves. Left ventricular function moderately impaired (ejection fraction 44 per cent).

QUESTIONS

1. What does this ECG show?
2. What is the mechanism of this?
3. What are the likely causes?
4. What are the key issues in managing this patient?

ECG ANALYSIS

Rate	66/min
Rhythm	Sinus rhythm with second-degree (Mobitz type II) atrioventricular block
QRS axis	Normal (+68°)
P waves	Normal
PR interval	140 ms (when P wave is followed by a QRS complex)
QRS duration	Normal (100 ms)
T waves	Normal
QTc interval	Normal (420 ms)

ANSWERS

1. Most of the P waves are followed by a QRS complex with a normal and constant PR interval, but every third P wave is not followed by QRS complex. This is **second-degree atrioventricular block of the Mobitz type II** type – there is intermittent failure of conduction of atrial impulses without a preceding lengthening of the PR interval.

2. Second-degree atrioventricular block (Mobitz type II) results from intermittent failure of conduction of atrial impulses through the atrioventricular node. Mobitz type II block is usually due to infranodal block (i.e. below the atrioventricular node, whereas in Mobitz type I block, the block is usually confined to the atrioventricular node itself).

3. Causes of Mobitz type II atrioventricular block include idiopathic fibrosis of conducting tissue, acute myocardial infarction and drug-related conduction problems.

4. A permanent pacemaker is indicated for chronic Mobitz type II atrioventricular block, whether symptomatic or asymptomatic.

COMMENTARY

- In Mobitz type II atrioventricular block:
  - the atrial rate is normally regular (but occasionally it is not).
  - the risk of Stokes–Adams attacks (a sudden, transient episode of syncope in which the patient becomes pale and collapses due to a temporary pause in cardiac rhythm) is high. The episode may be confused with epilepsy – the patient may lie for several minutes motionless, pale and pulseless, but there is no incontinence or abnormal movements and recovery to normality is quick, often with flushing afterwards. A permanent pacemaker is curative.
  - there is a risk of slow ventricular rate and sudden death.
- Mobitz type II atrioventricular block in acute infarction may progress unpredictably to complete heat block, so admission to a monitored area is mandatory:
  - in acute **inferior** infarction, ischaemia is usually transient and a full recovery can be expected – resolution can be expected in hours or days but occasionally it may take 2–3 weeks. Temporary pacing is rarely needed.
  - in acute **anterior** infarction, the combination of acute left ventricular dysfunction and a rhythm abnormality affects cardiac output markedly and mortality is increased considerably – temporary pacing may help increase cardiac output but does not alter outcome.

Further reading

Making Sense of the ECG 4th edition: Mobitz type II AV block, p 95.

Brignole M, Alboni P, Benditt DG *et al.* Guidelines on management (diagnosis and treatment) of syncope – update 2004. *Eur Heart J* 2004; **25**: 2054–72.

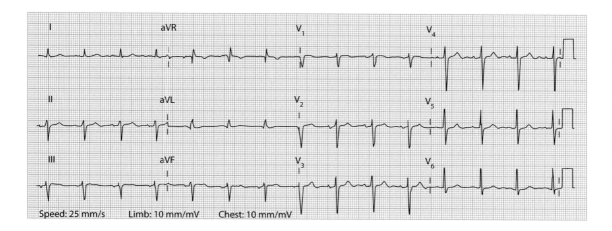

Speed: 25 mm/s   Limb: 10 mm/mV   Chest: 10 mm/mV

CLINICAL SCENARIO

Female, aged 78 years.

Presenting complaint
Asymptomatic – routine ECG performed prior to orthopaedic surgery (right total hip replacement).

History of presenting complaint
No cardiac history as asymptomatic.

Past medical history
Osteoarthritis of the right hip.
No prior cardiac history.

Examination
Patient walks with a stick.
Comfortable at rest.
Pulse: 86/min, regular.
Blood pressure: 136/78.
JVP: not elevated.
Heart sounds: normal.
Chest auscultation: unremarkable.
No peripheral oedema.

Investigations
FBC: Hb 12.8, WCC 6.7, platelets 178.
U&E: Na 138, K 3.8, urea 5.7, creatinine 91.
Chest X-ray: normal heart size, clear lung fields.

QUESTIONS

1. What does this ECG show?
2. What can cause this?
3. Is any treatment necessary?

ECG ANALYSIS

Rate	86/min
Rhythm	Sinus rhythm
QRS axis	Left axis deviation (−51°)
P waves	Normal
PR interval	Normal (160 ms)
QRS duration	Normal (90 ms)
T waves	Normal
QTc interval	Normal (450 ms)

ANSWERS

1. Left axis deviation (QRS axis −51°).
2. Left axis deviation can occur in normal individuals, and also as a result of:
   - left anterior hemiblock
   - inferior myocardial infarction
   - Wolff–Parkinson–White syndrome
   - ventricular tachycardia.
3. Left axis deviation does not require treatment in its own right.

COMMENTARY

- The normal QRS axis lies between −30° and +90° (although some cardiologists accept anything up to +120° as normal). Left axis deviation is conventionally diagnosed when the QRS axis lies more leftward (negative) than −30°.

- A quick way to assess QRS axis is to look at leads I and II:
  - If the QRS complex is positive in leads I and II, then the axis is normal.
  - If the QRS complex is positive in lead I and negative in lead II, then there is left axis deviation.
  - If the QRS complex is negative in lead I and positive in lead II, then there is right axis deviation.
  - Negative QRS complexes in both leads I and II most commonly indicate incorrect positioning of the limb electrodes – check electrode placement and repeat the ECG as appropriate.
- The left bundle branch divides into two sub-branches or fascicles – the left anterior fascicle and the left posterior fascicle. Block of the left anterior fascicle (left anterior fascicular block, also known as left anterior hemiblock) can occur as a result of fibrosis of the conducting system (of any cause) or from myocardial infarction.
- On its own, left anterior fascicular block is not thought to carry any prognostic significance and no specific treatment is required. The isolated presence of left axis deviation should not be a bar to orthopaedic surgery.

Further reading

Making Sense of the ECG 4th edition: The axis, p 105; Is there left axis deviation? p 114.

Meek S, Morri F. ABC of clinical electrocardiography: Introduction. I – Leads, rate, rhythm, and cardiac axis. *Br Med J* 2002; **324**: 415– 8.

CASE 24

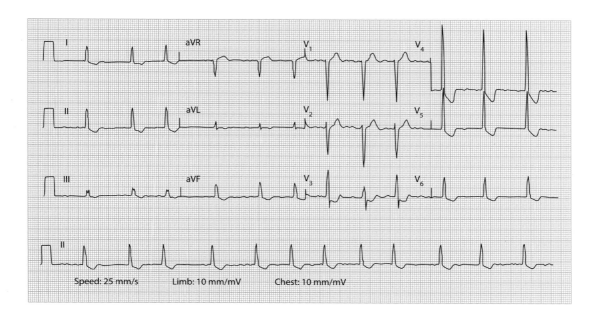

Speed: 25 mm/s   Limb: 10 mm/mV   Chest: 10 mm/mV

CLINICAL SCENARIO

Female, aged 80 years.

Presenting complaint

Nausea and vomiting.

History of presenting complaint

Patient has had atrial fibrillation for several years – not previously problematic. A week ago, felt generally unwell with mild fever and cough productive of green sputum. Family doctor prescribed antibiotics for a presumed respiratory tract infection. Although her symptoms were resolving, she stopped eating and drinking as she felt nauseous.

Past medical history

Rheumatic fever as child. Mixed mitral valve disease but symptoms not severe enough to warrant valve surgery. Under regular follow-up with a cardiologist.

Examination

Pulse: 72/min, irregularly irregular.
Blood pressure: 130/80.
JVP: not elevated.
Heart sounds: loud first heart sound; mid-diastolic rumble and pan-systolic murmur.
Chest auscultation: unremarkable.
Trace of ankle oedema.

Investigations

FBC: Hb 13.9, WCC 8.1, platelets 233.
U&E: Na 132, K 3.1, urea 8.9, creatinine 286.
Thyroid function: normal.
Troponin I: negative.
Chest X-ray: mild cardiomegaly.
Echocardiogram: thickened mitral leaflets with restricted movement; moderate mitral regurgitation into a moderately dilated left atrium. Left ventricular function moderately impaired (ejection fraction 43 per cent).

QUESTIONS

1. What does this ECG show?
2. Is this a sign of drug toxicity?

3. What mechanisms are involved?
4. What are the common ECG findings of digoxin toxicity?

ECG ANALYSIS

Rate	72/min
Rhythm	Atrial fibrillation
QRS axis	Normal (+47°)
P waves	Absent
PR interval	N/A
QRS duration	Normal (110 ms)
T waves	Inverted in most leads
QTc interval	Normal (440 ms)

Additional comments

There is downsloping 'reverse tick' ST segment depression in the inferior and anterolateral leads.

ANSWERS

1. The rhythm is irregularly irregular with no discernible P waves (atrial fibrillation). The QRS complexes are normal but the ST segments are downward-sloping with a 'reverse tick' morphology: this is typical (although not diagnostic) of **digitalis (digoxin) effect**.

2. It is important to distinguish between the effects of digoxin on the ECG at normal therapeutic levels, and the effects of digoxin toxicity. ST segment depression is a normal finding in patients on digoxin, as is a reduction in T wave size and shortening of the QT interval. At toxic levels of digoxin, T wave inversion can occur, as can virtually any arrhythmia (but classically paroxysmal atrial tachycardia with atrioventricular block).

3. The effects of digoxin on the ECG are complex. It has a direct action by inducing electrical and mechanical effects by inhibiting sodium ion (and secondarily potassium ion) transport across myocardial and pacemaker cells, and an indirect effect by increasing vagal tone.

4. The most common ECG findings of digoxin toxicity are: heart block, bradycardia, junctional tachycardia and atrial fibrillation. Risk of digoxin toxicity increases with renal impairment, concomitant prescribing with verapamil or amiodarone, dehydration and hypokalaemia. The half-life of digoxin with normal renal function is 36–48 h, so in toxicity simply stopping the drug and supportive measures may be enough. It may be as long as 5 days in renal impairment. Digoxin is not removed by dialysis – if toxicity causes arrhythmias or malignant hyperkalaemia (due to paralysed cell membrane-bound ATPase-dependent Na/K pumps), antibody fragments that bind with digoxin (Digibind) provide a specific antidote.

COMMENTARY

- As well as digoxin effect, other causes of ST segment depression include myocardial ischaemia, acute posterior myocardial infarction, reciprocal changes in acute ST segment elevation myocardial infarction, and left ventricular hypertrophy with 'strain'.
- Always be careful to distinguish between ECG features seen with normal digoxin levels and those indicative of digoxin toxicity. Digoxin levels can be measured and guide clinical decision making.
- Symptoms of digoxin toxicity are non-specific: blurred vision, impaired colour perception (yellow or green vision was first reported by William Withering in 1785), confusion, anorexia, nausea, vomiting and diarrhoea.
- The risk of digoxin toxicity depends on the dose of digoxin, physical size of the patient, renal function and potassium level. Levels do not need to be routinely monitored but they are helpful if toxicity is suspected.
- Caution – always interpret digoxin levels in the light of clinical and chemical data.

Further reading

Making Sense of the ECG 4th edition: Atrial fibrillation, p 59; Are the ST segments depressed? p 171; Digoxin and the ECG, p 175.

Rautaharju PM, Surawicz B, Gettes LS. AHA/ACCF/ HRS recommendations for the standardization and interpretation of the electrocardiogram: Part IV: The ST segment, T and U waves, and the QT interval. *J Am Coll Cardiol* 2009; **53**: 982–91.

CASE 25

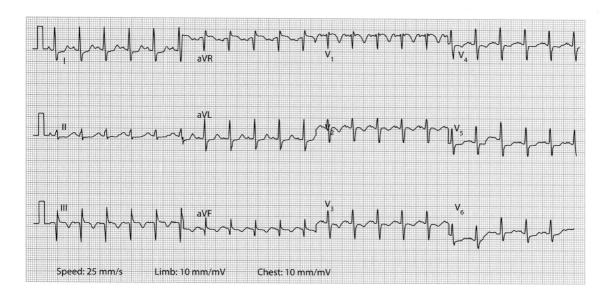

Speed: 25 mm/s   Limb: 10 mm/mV   Chest: 10 mm/mV

CLINICAL SCENARIO

Female, aged 72 years.

Presenting complaint

Sudden onset breathlessness and pleuritic chest pain.

History of presenting complaint

Patient underwent left total knee replacement 2 days ago. Developed sudden onset breathlessness and right-sided pleuritic chest pain.

Past medical history

Left knee osteoarthritis.

Examination

Patient breathless at rest. In discomfort.
Pulse: 128/min, regular.
Blood pressure: 116/84.
JVP: elevated by 3 cm.
Heart sounds: gallop rhythm.
Chest auscultation: pleural rub heard in right midzone.
No peripheral oedema.

Investigations

FBC: Hb 11.8, WCC 11.1, platelets 323.
U&E: Na 141, K 4.3, urea 5.4, creatinine 95.
Chest X-ray: normal heart size, clear lung fields.

QUESTIONS

1. What does this ECG show?
2. What is the likely cause of this ECG appearance?
3. What investigations would be appropriate?
4. What are the treatment options?

ECG ANALYSIS

Rate	128/min
Rhythm	Sinus tachycardia
QRS axis	Normal (+16°)
P waves	Normal
PR interval	Normal (160 ms)
QRS duration	Normal (84 ms)
T waves	Inverted in leads III, aVF, V1–V4
QTc interval	Mildly prolonged (467 ms)

Additional comments

There is an S1Q3T3 pattern and anterior T wave inversion.

ANSWERS

1. This ECG shows:
   - sinus tachycardia
   - an S wave in lead I, and a Q wave and an inverted T wave in lead III (S1Q3T3)
   - anterior T wave inversion.
2. Acute pulmonary embolism.
3. Appropriate investigations for suspected acute pulmonary embolism include:
   - arterial blood gases
   - D-dimers
   - chest X-ray (usually normal initially)
   - imaging studies: computed tomography (CT) pulmonary angiography or nuclear scintigraphy lung ventilation–perfusion (V/Q) scan.
4. The treatment of pulmonary embolism includes anticoagulation with heparin/warfarin, although consider thrombolysis in patients who have massive pulmonary embolism and/or are haemodynamically unstable. Administer oxygen therapy for hypoxia.

COMMENTARY

- Sinus tachycardia is the commonest ECG abnormality found in pulmonary embolism.
- ECG indicators of right heart strain (pressure and/or volume overload) include the S1Q3T3 pattern, also referred to as the McGinn-White sign (after Sylvester McGinn and Paul White, who first described the pattern in 1935). However, although the S1Q3T3 pattern is often described as an indicator of pulmonary embolism, it is relatively insensitive and non-specific – it is only evident in around half of patients, and can occur in any condition that causes acute right heart strain (e.g. bronchospasm, pneumothorax).
- In those patients already suspected of having a pulmonary embolism, the presence of anterior T wave inversion has a sensitivity and specificity of >80 per cent for diagnosing massive pulmonary embolism.
- Other ECG abnormalities seen in pulmonary embolism can include incomplete right bundle branch block, P pulmonale (right atrial enlargement), nonspecific ST segment changes and atrial fibrillation/flutter.
- A normal ECG does not exclude a diagnosis of pulmonary embolism.

Further reading

Making Sense of the ECG 4th edition: Sinus tachycardia, p 55; S1Q3T3 pattern, p 141.

Ferrari E, Imbert A, Chevalier T *et al*. The ECG in pulmonary embolism. Predictive value of negative T waves in precordial leads – 80 case reports. *Chest* 1997; **111**: 537–43.

McGinn S, White PD. Acute cor pulmonale resulting from pulmonary embolism. Its clinical recognition. *JAMA* 1935; **104**: 1473–80.

CASE 26

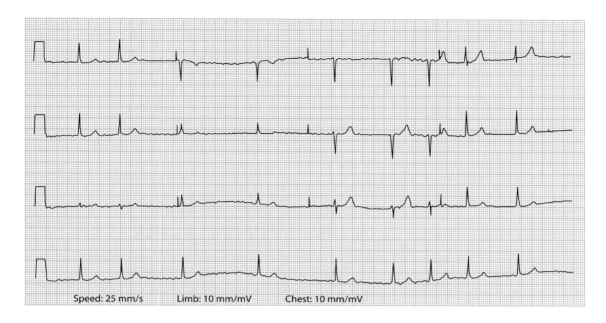

Speed: 25 mm/s   Limb: 10 mm/mV   Chest: 10 mm/mV

CLINICAL SCENARIO

Female, aged 69 years.

Presenting complaint
Breathless, especially going up stairs.

History of presenting complaint
Was fairly well until 3 months ago when a new family doctor changed her medication.

Past medical history
Rheumatic fever.
Mitral regurgitation.

Examination
Pulse: 54/min, irregularly irregular.
Blood pressure: 110/70.
JVP: elevated by 2 cm.

Heart sounds: loud first sound, mitral regurgitation easily heard.
Chest auscultation: unremarkable.
Mild pitting ankle oedema.

Investigations
FBC: Hb 12.6, WCC 5.9, platelets 345.
U&E: Na 133, K 4.1, urea 6.7, creatinine 168.
Thyroid function: normal.
Chest X-ray: mild cardiomegaly, early pulmonary congestion.
Echocardiogram: thickened mitral leaflets, moderate mitral regurgitation into a moderately dilated left atrium. Left ventricular function mildly impaired (ejection fraction 45 per cent).

QUESTIONS

1. What does this ECG show?
2. What is the mechanism of this?
3. What are the likely causes?

ECG ANALYSIS

Rate	54/min
Rhythm	Atrial fibrillation with a slow ventricular response
QRS axis	Normal (+31°)
P waves	Absent
PR interval	N/A
QRS duration	Normal (80 ms)
T waves	Normal
QTc interval	Normal (402 ms)

ANSWERS

1. This ECG shows an irregularly irregular rhythm with absent P waves and a slow ventricular rate: this is **atrial fibrillation with a slow ventricular response**.
2. Atrial fibrillation with a slow ventricular response is usually due to an inappropriately high dose of a rate-limiting drug (such as a beta blocker, rate-limiting calcium channel blocker or digoxin), although sometimes atrial fibrillation itself can occur with a relatively slow ventricular rate.
3. Many patients with atrial fibrillation are stable for years on their rate-controlling medication regimen but their ventricular rate control may be affected by:
   - intercurrent illness – may cause an increased heart rate, e.g. respiratory infection
   - drug compliance – failure to take as prescribed may cause inappropriately high or low drug levels
   - changing renal function with age – affects the levels of drugs that are renally excreted
   - gastrointestinal symptoms – may make absorption unpredictable
   - initiation of other medication – some may increase digoxin levels (amiodarone, diltiazem, verapamil, spironolactone); some may reduce levels (antacids, sulphasalazine, metoclopramide, domperidone).

In this case, the cause of the 'slow' atrial fibrillation was a change in digoxin dose from 125 mcg to 250 mcg daily, despite the impaired renal function.

COMMENTARY

- Always ensure that the rhythm has been diagnosed correctly before giving treatment – an inaccurate diagnosis means incorrect treatment that may cause symptoms to get worse.
- 'Slow' atrial fibrillation may not be easy to diagnose as the ECG baseline does not always show fibrillation waves and QRS complexes may look remarkably regular.
- Digoxin is renally excreted and has a half-life of 36–48 h. It has a narrow therapeutic 'window' and so caution must be taken in making dose adjustments in patients with renal impairment.
- The signs of digoxin toxicity include:
  - cardiovascular – bradycardia (<60/min), atrioventricular conduction block, supraventricular tachycardia, ventricular extrasystoles
  - central nervous system – dizziness, confusion, nightmares, hallucinations
  - visual – yellowing of vision, halo effect
  - gastrointestinal – anorexia, nausea, vomiting, diarrhoea, abdominal pain.

Further reading

Making Sense of the ECG 4th edition: Atrial fibrillation, p 59.

CASE 27

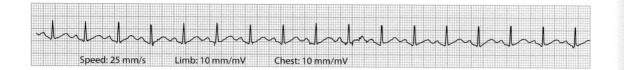

Speed: 25 mm/s   Limb: 10 mm/mV   Chest: 10 mm/mV

CLINICAL SCENARIO

Male, aged 57 years.

Presenting complaint
Sudden collapse.

History of presenting complaint
Patient admitted for investigation of right calf tenderness and swelling. Collapsed suddenly in the X-ray department immediately after he arrived for a leg ultrasound Doppler. This rhythm strip was recorded on arrival of the cardiac arrest team.

Past medical history
Patient had been resting at home following a right leg injury 3 weeks earlier.

Examination
Unresponsive – Glasgow Coma Scale score 3/15.
Pulse: unrecordable – pulses not palpable.
Blood pressure: unrecordable.
JVP: neck veins distended.
No respiratory movements.
Right calf red and swollen.

Investigations
FBC: Hb 14.1, WCC 10.6, platelets 306.
U&E: Na 137, K 4.1, urea 6.7, creatinine 112.
Chest X-ray: normal heart size, clear lung fields.

QUESTIONS

1. What does this ECG rhythm strip show?
2. What is the clinical diagnosis, and the likely underlying cause?
3. What action should be taken?

ECG ANALYSIS

Rate	108/min
Rhythm	Sinus tachycardia
QRS axis	Unable to assess (single lead)
P waves	Normal
PR interval	Normal (195 ms)
QRS duration	Normal (80 ms)
T waves	Normal
QTc interval	Mildly prolonged (456 ms)

ANSWERS

1. This ECG rhythm strips shows sinus tachycardia, 108/min.
2. The patient has collapsed and is unconscious (Glasgow Coma Scale score 3/15) with no detectable cardiac output. This is therefore a cardiac arrest with **pulseless electrical activity** (PEA), sometimes also called electromechanical dissociation (EMD). The likely cause in this clinical context is **massive pulmonary embolism**, secondary to a deep vein thrombosis of the right leg.
3. Follow standard basic and advanced life support algorithms. PEA is a non-shockable rhythm and it is particularly important to look for an underlying treatable cause.

COMMENTARY

- PEA occurs when the heart is still working electrically but is failing to produce an output.

- It is important to remember that PEA can be seen in conjunction with *any* cardiac rhythm that would normally sustain a circulation. The diagnosis of PEA is therefore not an ECG diagnosis *per se* (the ECG can look entirely normal), but is based upon the clinical context of a patient with no cardiac output despite a heart that appears to be working electrically.
- Causes of PEA include:
  - hypoxia
  - hypovolaemia
  - hyperkalaemia, hypokalaemia, hypocalcaemia, acidaemia, and other metabolic disorders
  - hypothermia
  - tension pneumothorax
  - tamponade
  - toxic substances
  - thromboembolism (pulmonary embolus/coronary thrombosis).
- PEA is managed according to the non-shockable rhythms (PEA and asystole) treatment algorithm of the Resuscitation Council (UK).

Further reading

Making Sense of the ECG 4th edition: How is the patient?, p 46; Adult Advanced Life Support guideline, p 85.

Resuscitation Council (UK). Resuscitation guidelines. 2010. Available at: www.resus.org.uk

CASE 28

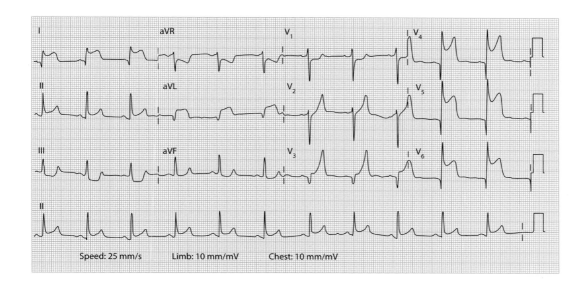

Speed: 25 mm/s   Limb: 10 mm/mV   Chest: 10 mm/mV

CLINICAL SCENARIO

Female, aged 76 years.

Presenting complaint
Woken from sleep with severe chest pain.

History of presenting complaint
Had angina on exertion for over 4 years. Similar pain to usual angina but much worse. Never had pain at rest or at night before – felt like there was 'someone sitting on my chest'. The pain radiated to the left arm and was associated with breathlessness. She was afraid she might die.

Past medical history
Hypertension – well controlled on amlodipine.
Diabetes mellitus.
Hypercholesterolaemia.
Ex-smoker. Strong family history of coronary artery disease.

Examination
Pulse: 66/min, regular.
Blood pressure: 182/98.
JVP: not elevated.
Heart sounds: soft pansystolic murmur at apex (mitral regurgitation).
Chest auscultation: bilateral basal crackles.
No peripheral oedema.

Investigations
FBC: Hb 11.5, WCC 5.2, platelets 401.
U&E: Na 132, K 4.5, urea 7.0, creatinine 131.
Troponin I: elevated at 12966 (after 6 h).
Chest X-ray: mild cardiomegaly, early pulmonary congestion.
Echocardiogram: mild mitral regurgitation. Left ventricular function mildly impaired (ejection fraction 47 per cent).

QUESTIONS

1. What does this ECG show?
2. What is the mechanism of this?
3. What are the likely causes?
4. What are the key issues in managing this patient?

ECG ANALYSIS

Rate	66/min
Rhythm	Sinus rhythm
QRS axis	Normal (+70°)
P waves	Normal
PR interval	Normal (160 ms)
QRS duration	Normal (96 ms)
T waves	Merged with ST segment
QTc interval	Normal (420 ms)

Additional comments

There is ST segment elevation in the lateral leads (I, aVL, V4–V6).

ANSWERS

1. There is ST segment elevation in limb leads I and aVL and chest leads V4–V6. This is an **acute lateral ST segment elevation myocardial infarction** (STEMI).
2. Acute occlusion of the circumflex coronary artery.
3. A previously stable coronary endothelial plaque has ruptured, exposing the lipid-rich core. Platelets adhere, change shape and secrete adenosine diphosphate (ADP) and other pro-aggregants. These seal and stabilize the plaque but at the cost of narrowing of the coronary artery lumen. This is often totally, or almost totally, occluded.
4. Treatment is aimed at restoring coronary patency. This can be achieved by:
   - primary percutaneous coronary intervention (PCI) in the catheter laboratory
   - thrombolysis, using an intravenous thrombolytic to break down the thrombus and reopen the occluded coronary artery.

   Immediate management also includes pain relief (opiates plus an anti-emetic) and anti-platelet therapy (aspirin with clopidogrel).

Admit the patient to a monitored area to treat any complications (heart failure, potentially lethal arrhythmia). Commence secondary prevention (angiotensin-converting enzyme (ACE) inhibitor, beta blocker, statin and anti-smoking advice). Remember to provide primary prevention advice to family members.

COMMENTARY

- An urgent ECG is required in any patient presenting with cardiac-sounding chest pain. The presence of ST segment elevation signifies acute occlusion of a coronary artery and indicates a need for urgent restoration of coronary blood flow (reperfusion). This can be achieved with primary PCI or, if primary PCI is unavailable, with thrombolysis. Time is of the essence – the longer reperfusion is delayed, the more myocardial necrosis will occur.
- If thrombolysis is administered, a failure to achieve coronary reperfusion may indicate the need to consider repeat thrombolysis or coronary angiography and 'rescue' PCI. If the ST segment elevation has not fallen by ≥50 per cent 2 h after the start of thrombolysis, there is an 80–85 per cent probability that normal coronary blood flow has not been restored.
- The differential diagnosis of ST segment elevation includes acute myocardial infarction, left ventricular aneurysm, Prinzmetal's (vasospastic) angina, pericarditis, high take-off, left bundle branch block and Brugada syndrome.

Further reading

Making Sense of the ECG 4th edition: Are the ST segments elevated?, p 159; ST segment elevation myocardial infarction, p 160.

Rautaharju PM, Surawicz B, Gettes LS. AHA/ACCF/ HRS recommendations for the standardization and interpretation of the electrocardiogram: Part IV: The ST segment, T and U waves, and the QT interval. *J Am Coll Cardiol* 2009; **53**: 982–91.

CASE 29

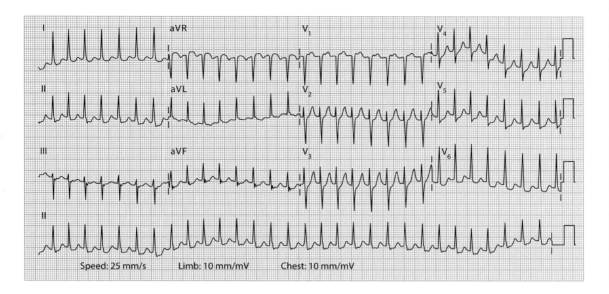

Speed: 25 mm/s   Limb: 10 mm/mV   Chest: 10 mm/mV

CLINICAL SCENARIO

Female, aged 23 years.

Presenting complaint
Rapid regular palpitations.

History of presenting complaint
Two-year history of episodic rapid regular palpitations, normally lasting only a few minutes, with a sudden onset and termination. The current episode started suddenly 2 h prior to presentation.

Past medical history
Nil.

Examination
Pulse: 180/min, regular.
Blood pressure: 112/72.
JVP: normal.
Heart sounds: normal (tachycardic).
Chest auscultation: unremarkable.

Investigations
FBC: Hb 13.5, WCC 5.2, platelets 302.
U&E: Na 140, K 4.4, urea 4.5, creatinine 73.
Chest X-ray: normal heart size, clear lung fields.

QUESTIONS

1. What does this ECG show?
2. What is the underlying pathophysiological mechanism?
3. What initial treatment would be appropriate?
4. What treatment might be appropriate in the longer term?

ECG ANALYSIS

Rate	180/min
Rhythm	Atrioventricular nodal re-entry tachycardia
QRS axis	Normal (+22°)
P waves	Visible as a small negative deflection at the end of the QRS complex in the inferior leads
PR interval	Not applicable
QRS duration	Normal (60 ms)
T waves	Normal
QTc interval	Normal (450 ms)

ANSWERS

1. Atrioventricular nodal re-entry tachycardia (AVNRT).
2. A re-entry circuit involving a dual atrioventricular nodal pathway – one of the atrioventricular nodal pathways conducts impulses quickly (the 'fast' pathway) but has a long refractory period, the other pathway conducts impulses more slowly (the 'slow' pathway) but has a shorter refractory period (see Commentary).
3. Transiently blocking the atrioventricular node can terminate the AVNRT. Methods to achieve this include:
   - Valsalva manoeuvre
   - carotid sinus massage
   - intravenous adenosine
   - intravenous verapamil.
4. The patient can be taught the Valsalva manoeuvre to try to terminate episodes. Recurrent AVNRT may require treatment with anti-arrhythmic drugs (e.g. verapamil, propranolol, digoxin) or an electrophysiological study with a view to a radiofrequency ablation procedure.

COMMENTARY

- In patients with a dual atrioventricular nodal pathway, an impulse arriving at the atrioventricular node will normally split and travel down both pathways at the same time, but the impulse travelling via the fast pathway arrives at the bundle of His first and depolarizes the ventricles. By the time the impulse travelling down the slow pathway arrives at the bundle of His, the bundle is refractory and so this impulse goes no further.
- However, if a supraventricular ectopic beat happens to occur during the refractory period of the fast pathway, this ectopic will travel down the slow pathway and, by the time it reaches the end of the slow pathway, the fast pathway may have repolarized. If so, this impulse will then travel back *up* along the fast pathway, and then back down the slow pathway, ad infinitum. In the common form of AVNRT, this slow-fast re-entry circuit gives rise to the arrhythmia. Fast-slow and slow-slow re-entry circuits are also possible.
- In AVNRT, P waves are often hard or even impossible to discern. In around a quarter of cases, they are hidden within the QRS complexes. In another two-thirds of cases, they can be seen as a small negative deflection at the end of the QRS complexes in the inferior leads, and/or as a small positive deflection at the end of the QRS complex in lead V1. In a small number of cases, the P wave can be found just before the QRS complex.
- AVNRT is around 10 times commoner than atrioventricular re-entry tachycardia (AVRT – the result of an atrioventricular accessory pathway as seen in Wolff–Parkinson–White [WPW] syndrome). The ECG performed during sinus rhythm in a patient prone to AVNRT is usually normal, but in those prone to AVRT an ECG in sinus rhythm may reveal a short PR interval or delta wave, suggesting WPW syndrome. The distinction between AVRT and AVNRT can be difficult, however, and may require electrophysiological studies.

Further reading

Making Sense of the ECG 4th edition: Atrioventricular nodal re-entry tachycardia, p 73.

Katritsis DG, Camm AJ. Atrioventricular nodal reentrant tachycardia. *Circulation* 2010; **122**: 831–40.

Whinnett ZI, Sohaib SMA, Davies DW. Diagnosis and management of supraventricular tachycardia. *BMJ* 2012; **345**: e7769.

CASE 30

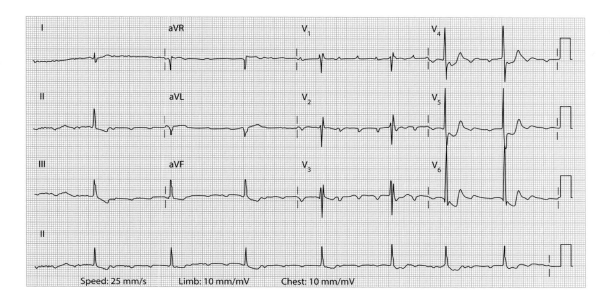

Speed: 25 mm/s   Limb: 10 mm/mV   Chest: 10 mm/mV

CLINICAL SCENARIO

Male, aged 84 years.

Presenting complaint
Increasing exertional breathlessness.

History of presenting complaint
Had been fairly well until developed chest infection. Breathlessness has got progressively worse since.

Past medical history
Previous rheumatic fever.

Examination
Pulse: 42/min, irregular.
Blood pressure: 122/76.
JVP: normal.
Heart sounds: normal.
Chest auscultation: unremarkable.
No peripheral oedema.

Investigations
FBC: Hb 11.1, WCC 4.7, platelets 224.
U&E: Na 135, K 4.7, urea 5.8, creatinine 146.
Thyroid function: normal.
Troponin I: negative.

QUESTIONS

1. What does this ECG show?
2. What is the mechanism of this?
3. What are the likely causes?
4. What are the key issues in managing this patient?

ECG ANALYSIS

Rate	42/min
Rhythm	Atrial tachycardia with variable atrioventricular block
QRS axis	Normal (+80°)
P waves	Present but abnormal morphology
PR interval	N/A
QRS duration	Normal (80 ms)
T waves	Abnormal
QTc interval	Normal (350 ms)

Additional comments

The P waves are abnormally shaped, indicating an atrial focus away from the sinoatrial node, and the P wave rate is 156/min (but most P waves are not conducted to the ventricles). There is also a partial RBBB pattern and lateral ST segment depression.

ANSWERS

1. This ECG shows regular P waves at a rate of 156/min. The P waves have an abnormal morphology, indicating a focus away from the sinoatrial node. Only some of the P waves are followed by QRS complexes, and the QRS rate is variable. This is **atrial tachycardia with variable atrioventricular block**.

2. Atrial tachycardia results from increased automaticity of a focus of depolarization in the atria. The variable atrioventricular block is due to depressed conduction through the atrioventricular node.

3. The presence of 'reverse tick' lateral ST segment depression suggests that the patient is taking digoxin, and indeed this arrhythmia proved to be the result of digoxin toxicity.

4. Temporary (and occasionally permanent) withdrawal of digoxin treatment. Supportive measures until digoxin levels have fallen to therapeutic levels. An alternative anti-arrhythmic drug may be required.

COMMENTARY

- In atrial tachycardia, the ventricular rate depends upon the degree of atrioventricular block. With 1:1 conduction, the ventricular rate may be rapid.
- Atrial tachycardia may occur in tachy-brady syndrome, rheumatic and ischaemic heart disease, chronic airways disease and cardiomyopathy.
- Digoxin affects the heart in various ways:
  - an inotropic effect through inhibition of the sodium/potassium/ATPase pump
  - increased automaticity of Purkinje fibres
  - slowing of conduction through the atrioventricular node due to increased vagal activity.
- With digoxin toxicity, increased automaticity results in an increased atrial rate and slowing of conduction induces atrioventricular block and subsequent slowing of the ventricular rate.
- Toxicity can occur with digoxin levels within the therapeutic range if there is severe hypokalaemia (often due to diuretic therapy) or renal impairment.
- Although paroxysmal atrial tachycardia with variable block is considered the 'hallmark' of digoxin toxicity, in clinical practice the arrhythmia is often sustained. In addition, digoxin can cause almost any cardiac arrhythmia.

Further reading

Making Sense of the ECG 4th edition: Atrial tachycardia, p 66; Effects of digoxin on the ECG, p 175.

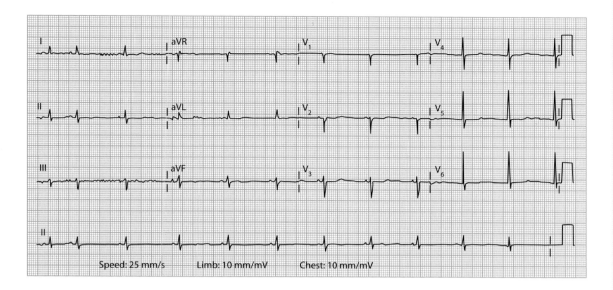

Speed: 25 mm/s   Limb: 10 mm/mV   Chest: 10 mm/mV

CLINICAL SCENARIO

Male, aged 29 years.

Presenting complaint
Episodic palpitations.

History of presenting complaint
A 2-year history of rapid regular palpitations, occurring once a week on average and lasting for between 10 and 60 minutes. Prolonged episodes are associated with dizziness.

Past medical history
Nil.

Examination
Pulse: 66/min, regular with infrequent ectopics.
Blood pressure: 132/82.
JVP: not elevated.
Heart sounds: normal.
Chest auscultation: unremarkable.
No peripheral oedema.

Investigations
FBC: Hb 14.5, WCC 5.7, platelets 286.
U&E: Na 141, K 4.6, urea 4.1, creatinine 72.
Thyroid function: normal.
Chest X-ray: normal heart size, clear lung fields.

QUESTIONS

1. What does this ECG show?
2. What is the likely cause of the patient's palpitations?
3. What further investigations would be appropriate?

ECG ANALYSIS

Rate	66/min
Rhythm	Sinus rhythm with a single supraventricular ectopic beat
QRS axis	Normal (+0°)
P waves	Normal
PR interval	Short (100 ms)
QRS duration	Normal (76 ms)
T waves	Normal
QTc interval	Normal (450 ms)

Additional comments

The PR interval is short at 100 ms.

ANSWERS

1. The ECG shows a short PR interval, measuring 100 ms (2.5 small squares). In the context of episodic palpitations, this is suggestive of a diagnosis of Lown–Ganong–Levine (LGL) syndrome. The diagnosis can be confirmed by demonstrating the occurrence of episodes of atrioventricular re-entry tachycardia (AVRT).
2. The presence of an accessory pathway in LGL syndrome allows for an atrioventricular re-entry tachycardia.
3. The patient's ECG should be recorded during an episode of palpitation in order to make a diagnosis of AVRT and thus to confirm LGL syndrome. Ambulatory ECG recording can be used. As the patient's symptoms are occurring once a week on average, a 7-day ECG event recorder or a Cardiomemo would be the most effective ways of trying to capture an event.

COMMENTARY

- The diagnosis of LGL syndrome requires the presence of a short PR interval (<120 ms), a normal QRS complex duration and episodes of AVRT.
- The presence of a short PR interval *in the absence* of any history of palpitations is not sufficient for a diagnosis of LGL syndrome, and may indicate a normal variant of accelerated conduction through the atrioventricular node rather than the presence of an accessory pathway.
- LGL syndrome has often been described as being due to an accessory pathway that connects the atria to the bundle of His. Although several such pathways have been identified, such as James fibres, no single anatomical substrate specific to LGL syndrome has been found. The anatomical basis of LGL syndrome has therefore been the subject of debate, with many questioning whether it is a specific entity in its own right or whether it is simply a clinical manifestation of a range of different atrioventricular conduction anomalies.

Further reading

Making Sense of the ECG 4th edition: Lown–Ganong–Levine syndrome, p 129.

Lown B, Ganong WF, Levine SA. The syndrome of short P-R interval, normal QRS complex and paroxysmal rapid heart action. *Circulation* 1952; **5:** 693.

CASE 32

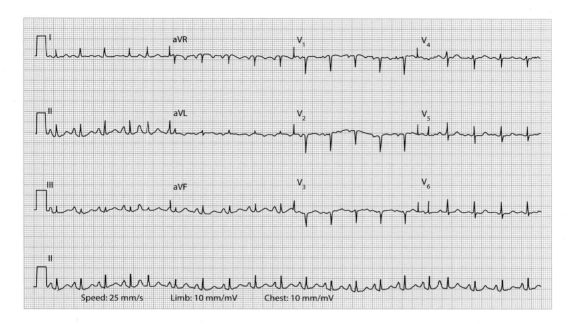

Speed: 25 mm/s   Limb: 10 mm/mV   Chest: 10 mm/mV

CLINICAL SCENARIO

Male, aged 74 years.

Presenting complaint
Admitted to hospital with chest pain and breathlessness on exertion.

History of presenting complaint
Symptom-free until 3 months ago. Developed chest pain on exertion, especially if walking uphill, in cold weather or when wind blowing. Occasionally had chest pain at rest, requiring glyceryl trinitrate spray. Pain was gradually getting worse. Had one episode of chest pain that woke him the night before admission.

Past medical history
History of hypertension and hypercholesterolaemia. Acute myocardial infarction 3 years ago, treated with thrombolysis.
Chronic bronchitis on home nebulizers.

Examination
Pulse: 120/min, regular with occasional ectopic beats.
JVP: not elevated.
Heart sounds: soft ejection systolic murmur in aortic area, radiating to neck.
Chest auscultation: unremarkable.
No peripheral oedema.

Investigations
FBC: Hb 12.9, WCC 6.5, platelets 342.
U&E: Na 136, K 4.7, urea 5.1, creatinine 132.
Troponin I: negative.
Chest X-ray: mild cardiomegaly, early pulmonary congestion.
Echocardiogram: mild aortic stenosis, with pressure drop of 20 mmHg across valve, mild mitral regurgitation into a non-dilated left atrium. Left ventricular function moderately impaired (ejection fraction 43 per cent) with anterior wall akinesia.

QUESTIONS

1. What does this ECG show?
2. What is the mechanism of this?
3. What are the likely causes?
4. What are the key issues in managing this patient?

ECG ANALYSIS

Rate	120/min
Rhythm	Sinus tachycardia with occasional atrial ectopic beats
QRS axis	Normal (+53°)
P waves	Normal
PR interval	Normal (180 ms)
QRS duration	Normal (80 ms)
T waves	Normal
QTc interval	Normal (440 ms)

Additional comments

Anterior Q waves (leads V1–V3).

ANSWERS

1. There are Q waves in the anterior chest leads V1–V3, indicative of a previous anterior myocardial infarction. Q waves are considered 'pathological' if they exceed two small squares in depth, or are greater than 25 per cent of the size of the following R wave, and/or are greater than 1 small square wide.
2. Previous acute occlusion of the left anterior descending coronary artery.
3. Rupture of coronary atheroma, platelet activation and thrombus formation. Thrombolysis may restore coronary patency by dissolving thrombus overlying a ruptured coronary plaque but does not affect the size of the underlying coronary plaque. With progression of atheromatous deposition despite secondary preventive measures, flow past the coronary plaque slowly declines until physical activity leads to an imbalance between myocardial demand and supply and consequently the onset of symptoms.
4. If symptomatic, investigate for evidence of coronary artery disease – consider, as appropriate, functional imaging for ischaemia (stress echocardiogram, stress cardiac MRI scan or nuclear myocardial perfusion scan) or anatomical imaging for coronary atheroma (CT or invasive coronary angiography). In patients with known coronary artery disease, exercise treadmill testing can provide useful prognostic information. Consider secondary prevention (aspirin, clopidogrel, beta blocker, statin, angiotensin-converting enzyme (ACE) inhibitor) for all patients with a previous history of myocardial infarction.

COMMENTARY

- This patient clearly has a history of coronary artery disease, in view of the previous myocardial infarction, and presents with a clinical history consistent with unstable angina (ischaemic-sounding chest pain at rest but a negative troponin).
- A patient referred for 'routine' surgery may report a previous myocardial infarction or an ECG may show evidence of an 'old' (previously undiagnosed) myocardial infarction. The risk of an adverse perioperative event is increased with:
  - known coronary disease, especially within 3 months of a myocardial infarction
  - previously unidentified coronary disease
  - valvular heart disease, especially aortic stenosis
  - cardiac arrhythmia
  - heart failure/cardiogenic shock
  - coronary risk factors indicating high risk of coronary disease
  - renal impairment
  - abnormal liver function
  - previous stroke or transient ischaemic attack (TIA)
  - poor exercise tolerance.
- Guidelines are available to assess perioperative risk (see Further reading).

Further reading

Making Sense of the ECG 4th edition: The Q wave, p 139.
Poldermans D, Bax JJ, Boersma E *et al.* Guidelines for preoperative cardiac risk assessment and perioperative cardiac management in non-cardiac surgery. *Eur Heart J* 2009; **30**: 2769–812.

CASE 33

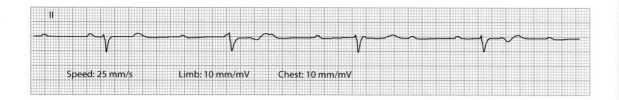

Speed: 25 mm/s   Limb: 10 mm/mV   Chest: 10 mm/mV

CLINICAL SCENARIO

Female, aged 86 years.

Presenting complaint
Dizziness and syncope, breathlessness.

History of presenting complaint
Four-day history of increasing breathlessness and dizziness, culminating in an episode of syncope in which the patient suddenly fell to the floor with little warning.

Past medical history
Myocardial infarction 2 months earlier.
Type 2 diabetes mellitus.

Examination
Pulse: 32/min, regular.
Blood pressure: 108/60.
JVP: elevated by 2 cm, intermittent cannon waves.
Heart sounds: variable intensity of second heart sound.
Chest auscultation: few bi-basal inspiratory crackles.
Mild peripheral oedema.

Investigations
FBC: Hb 12.1, WCC 6.3, platelets 206.
U&E: Na 136, K 4.2, urea 4.8, creatinine 81.
Thyroid function: normal.
Chest X-ray: cardiomegaly, pulmonary vascular congestion.

QUESTIONS

1. What does this ECG show?
2. What are the possible causes?
3. What treatment is required?

ECG ANALYSIS

Rate	Atrial – 90/min Ventricular – 32/min
Rhythm	Third-degree atrioventricular block ('complete heart block')
QRS axis	Can't be measured (single lead)
P waves	Present
PR interval	Variable – no apparent connection between P waves and QRS complexes
QRS duration	Prolonged (140 ms)
T waves	Inverted in leads III, aVF, V1–V4
QTc interval	Prolonged (475 ms)

ANSWERS

1. Third-degree atrioventricular (AV) block ('complete heart block').
2. Third-degree AV block can result from:
   - ischaemic heart disease
   - fibrosis and calcification of the conduction system (Lev's disease)
   - drugs that block the AV node (e.g. beta blockers, calcium channel blockers, digoxin – especially in combination)
   - Lyme disease
   - acute rheumatic fever
   - congenital complete heart block.
3. Third-degree AV block requires pacing if it is chronic and symptomatic (class I indication). Most authorities would also support pacing in asymptomatic patients with acquired third-degree AV block (class IIa indication).

COMMENTARY

- In third-degree AV block ('complete heart block'), there is complete interruption of conduction between atria and ventricles, so that the two are working independently. The atrial (P wave) rate is faster than the ventricular (QRS complex) rate, and the P waves bear no relationship to the QRS complexes.
- QRS complexes usually arise as the result of a ventricular escape rhythm. The QRS complexes are usually broad due to a subsidiary pacemaker ('escape rhythm') arising in the left or right bundle branches. However, if the AV block occurs high up in the conduction system (at the level of the AV node) and a subsidiary pacemaker arises in the bundle of His, the QRS complexes may be narrow.
- Any atrial rhythm can coexist with third-degree AV block, and so the P waves may be abnormal or even absent.
- In a patient with a recent onset of third-degree AV block, always consider the possibility of Lyme disease. This is transmitted by the spirochaete *Borrelia burgdorferi* and, in the second stage of the illness, can lead to first-degree, second-degree or third-degree AV block. The AV block can resolve entirely in response to antibiotics, although the patient may require support with a temporary pacemaker during treatment.
- In congenital third-degree AV block, which is uncommon, the block is usually at the level of the AV node and is often associated with maternal anti-Ro or anti-La antibodies.

Further reading

Making Sense of the ECG 4th edition: Third-degree atrioventricular block, p 96; Pacemakers and implantable cardioverter defibrillators, p 209.

Epstein AE, DiMarco JP, Ellenbogen KA *et al.* ACC/AHA/HRS 2008 guidelines for device-based therapy of cardiac rhythm abnormalities. A Report of the American College of Cardiology/American Heart Association task force on practice guidelines (writing committee to revise the ACC/AHA/NASPE 2002 guideline update for implantation of cardiac pacemakers and antiarrhythmia devices). *J Am Coll Cardiol* 2008; **51**: e1–62.

The Task Force for Cardiac Pacing and Cardiac Resynchronization Therapy of the European Society of Cardiology (ESC.). 2013 ESC guidelines on cardiac pacing and cardiac resynchronization therapy. *Eur Heart J* 2013; **34**: 2281–329.

CASE 34

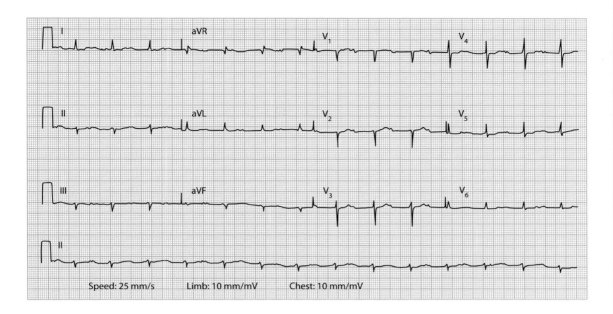

Speed: 25 mm/s   Limb: 10 mm/mV   Chest: 10 mm/mV

CLINICAL SCENARIO

Male, aged 69 years.

Presenting complaint
Feeling generally weak and lethargic. Also had frequent palpitations.

History of presenting complaint
Fit and well until about 3 months ago when diagnosed with hypertension and commenced on a thiazide-like diuretic.

Past medical history
Hypertension.

Examination
Pulse: 84/min, regular.
Blood pressure: 136/88.
JVP: normal.
Heart sounds: normal.
Chest auscultation: unremarkable.
No peripheral oedema.

Investigations
FBC: Hb 14.7, WCC 5.6, platelets 168.
U&E: Na 136, K 2.8, urea 4.6, creatinine 76.
Thyroid function: normal.
Chest X-ray: normal heart size, clear lung fields.
Echocardiogram: normal valves. Concentric left ventricular hypertrophy.

QUESTIONS

1. What does this ECG show?
2. What is the mechanism of this?
3. What are the likely causes?
4. What are the key issues in managing this patient?

ECG ANALYSIS

Rate	84/min
Rhythm	Sinus rhythm
QRS axis	Borderline left axis deviation (−30°)
P waves	Small but normal morphology
PR interval	Prolonged (400 ms)
QRS duration	Normal (80 ms)
T waves	Normal
QTc interval	Normal (390 ms)

ANSWERS

1. This ECG shows first-degree atrioventricular block (long PR interval), small T waves and there are U waves evident. These findings are secondary to **hypokalaemia**.

2. Depolarization of myocardial cells is dependent on the movement of ions across the cell membrane, the most important being potassium. The resting transmembrane potential is determined largely by the ratio of the intracellular (140 mmol/L) to extracellular (3.5 to 5 mmol/L) potassium ion concentration, and the absolute level of extracellular potassium ion concentration is the most important factor affecting the cell membrane.

3. Diuretic therapy, vomiting and diarrhoea, excessive perspiration, rectal villous adenoma, intestinal fistula, Cushing's and Conn's syndromes, alkalosis, purgative and laxative misuse, renal tubular failure, hypomagnesaemia (usually evident when K^+ remains low after potassium supplementation). Rare causes include Bartter's syndrome (hereditary defect of muscular ion channels) and hypokalaemic periodic paralysis.

4. If hypokalaemia is suspected, assess the patient for symptoms (such as muscle weakness and cramps) and enquire about prescribed drugs (diuretics are a common cause). Mild hypokalaemia can be corrected with dietary or oral supplements. Severe hypokalaemia is a medical emergency and should be corrected with slow intravenous infusion of appropriately diluted potassium chloride via a central line – fast or concentrated infusions may predispose to ventricular tachycardia.

COMMENTARY

- Mild hypokalaemia may occur without symptoms. Moderate hypokalaemia may cause muscle weakness, cramps and constipation. With more severe hypokalaemia, flaccid paralysis, hyporeflexia, respiratory depression and tetany may be seen.
- Hypokalaemia is much more common than hyperkalaemia and can produce the following ECG changes:
  - ST segment depression
  - decreased T wave amplitude
  - increased U wave amplitude
  - less commonly (and more subtly) prolonged QRS duration and increased P wave amplitude and duration.
- Resulting instability of cell membranes causes an increased risk of cardiac arrhythmia, especially atrial and ventricular ectopic beats, atrial and ventricular tachycardia, various heart blocks and ventricular fibrillation.
- Hypomagnesaemia is common with hypokalaemia; alone, it causes similar ECG abnormalities. Hypokalaemia is often difficult to correct until the magnesium level is normal.
- Caution – digoxin toxicity is more likely with hypokalaemia.
- It is important to measure serum potassium in all cases of suspected myocardial infarction. Although distinct changes may be observed, the ECG is not a reliable indicator of the serum potassium level.

Further reading

Making Sense of the ECG 4th edition: Hypokalaemia, p 200; Do the U waves appear too prominent? p 200.

CASE 35

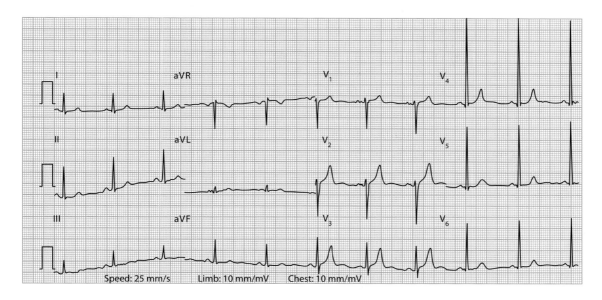

Speed: 25 mm/s   Limb: 10 mm/mV   Chest: 10 mm/mV

CLINICAL SCENARIO

Male, aged 48 years.

Presenting complaint
Asymptomatic – routine ECG performed during hypertension follow-up visit.

History of presenting complaint
Six-year history of hypertension, treated with an angiotensin-converting enzyme (ACE) inhibitor.

Past medical history
Six-year history of hypertension.

Examination
Patient comfortable at rest.
Pulse: 66/min, regular.
Blood pressure: 168/104.
JVP: not elevated.
Precordium: left parasternal heave.
Heart sounds: loud aortic component of second heart sound (A_2).
Chest auscultation: unremarkable.
No peripheral oedema.

Investigations
FBC: Hb 15.8, WCC 7.0, platelets 314.
U&E: Na 140, K 4.4, urea 6.2, creatinine 101.
Chest X-ray: normal heart size, clear lung fields.

QUESTIONS

1. What does this ECG show?
2. What investigation would help to confirm this?
3. What can cause these appearances? What is the likely cause here?
4. What are the treatment options?

ECG ANALYSIS

Rate	66/min
Rhythm	Sinus rhythm
QRS axis	Normal (+48°)
P waves	Normal
PR interval	Normal (167 ms)
QRS duration	Normal (96 ms)
T waves	Normal
QTc interval	Normal (420 ms)

Additional comments

In the chest leads there are deep S waves (up to 15 mm in lead V2) and tall R waves (up to 39 mm) in lead V4.

ANSWERS

1. This ECG shows deep S waves (up to 15 mm in lead V2) and tall R waves (up to 39 mm) in lead V4 in the chest leads. These appearances are indicative of left ventricular hypertrophy. The diagnostic criteria in this case include:
   - R wave in lead V4 measuring 39 mm
   - S wave in lead V1 plus R wave in lead V5 totalling 41 mm
   - Tallest R wave and deepest S wave in chest leads totalling 54 mm.
2. An echocardiogram (or cardiac magnetic resonance scan) would allow direct visualization of the left ventricle, assessment of the extent of left ventricular hypertrophy, assessment of left ventricular systolic (and diastolic) function, and also assessment of the heart valves.
3. Left ventricular hypertrophy can result from:
   - hypertension
   - aortic stenosis
   - coarctation of the aorta
   - hypertrophic cardiomyopathy.

   The clinical findings indicate that poorly controlled hypertension is the most likely cause of left ventricular hypertrophy in this case.
4. Where left ventricular hypertrophy is secondary to pressure overload of the left ventricle, the

appropriate treatment is that of the underlying cause – in this case, hypertension. The aim in most patients is to control the blood pressure to a level below 140/90.

COMMENTARY

- There are many criteria for the ECG diagnosis of left ventricular hypertrophy, with varying sensitivity and specificity. Generally, the diagnostic criteria are quite specific (if the criteria are present, the likelihood of the patient having left ventricular hypertrophy is >90 per cent), but not very sensitive (the criteria will fail to detect 40–80 per cent of patients with left ventricular hypertrophy). The diagnostic criteria include:
  - In the limb leads:
    – R wave greater than 11 mm in lead aVL
    – R wave greater than 20 mm in lead aVF
    – S wave greater than 14 mm in lead aVR
    – sum of R wave in lead I and S wave in lead III greater than 25 mm.
  - In the chest leads:
    – R wave of 25 mm or more in the left chest leads
    – S wave of 25 mm or more in the right chest leads
    – sum of S wave in lead V1 and R wave in lead V5 or V6 greater than 35 mm (Sokolow–Lyon criteria)
    – sum of tallest R wave and deepest S wave in the chest leads greater than 45 mm.
- The **Cornell criteria** involve measuring S wave in lead V3 and the R wave in lead aVL. Left ventricular hypertrophy is indicated by a sum of >28 mm in men and >20 mm in women.
- The **Romhilt–Estes scoring system** allocates points for the presence of certain criteria. A score of 5 indicates left ventricular hypertrophy and a score of 4 indicates probable left ventricular hypertrophy. Points are allocated as follows:
  - 3 points for (a) R or S wave in limb leads of 20 mm or more, (b) S wave in right chest leads of 25 mm or more, or (c) R wave in left chest leads of 25 mm or more

- 3 points for ST segment and T wave changes ('typical strain') in a patient not taking digitalis (1 point with digitalis)
- 3 points for P terminal force in V1 greater than 1 mm deep with a duration greater than 0.04 s
- 2 points for left axis deviation (beyond – 15 degrees)
- 1 point for QRS complex duration greater than 0.09 s

- 1 point for intrinsicoid deflection (the interval from the start of the QRS complex to the peak of the R wave) in V5 or V6 greater than 0.05 s.

Further reading

Making Sense of the ECG 4th edition: Left ventricular hypertrophy, p 146.

Bauml MA, Underwood DA. Left ventricular hypertrophy: An overlooked cardiovascular risk factor. *Cleveland Clinic J Med* 2010; **77**: 381–7.

CASE 36

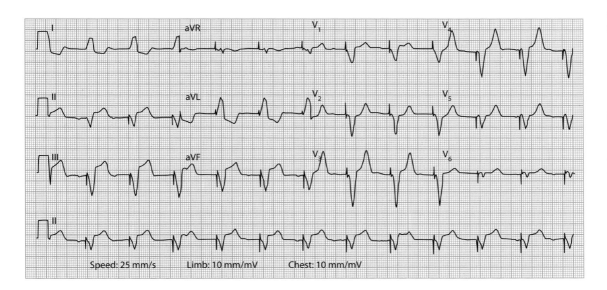

Speed: 25 mm/s   Limb: 10 mm/mV   Chest: 10 mm/mV

CLINICAL SCENARIO

Female, aged 79 years.

Presenting complaint

Breathlessness on exertion.

History of presenting complaint

Patient has had episodes of syncope and breathlessness for months. The syncope resolved following treatment but her breathlessness never improved back to normal. She now has episodes of paroxysmal nocturnal dyspnoea. As she attends the hospital regularly, she reported her persistent symptoms to the cardiac physiologist.

Past medical history

Congestive cardiac failure – unsure of medication but been on escalating doses of several drugs since she developed breathlessness.

Examination

Pulse: 72/min, regular.
Blood pressure: 126/98.
JVP: elevated by 2 cm.
Heart sounds: systolic murmur 3/6 in mitral area.
Chest auscultation: unremarkable.
Mild pitting ankle oedema.

Investigations

FBC: Hb 11.6, WCC 4.2, platelets 176.
U&E: Na 133, K 4.3, urea 8.5, creatinine 234.
Chest X-ray: marked cardiomegaly, fluid in horizontal fissure.
Echocardiogram: moderate mitral regurgitation into a moderately dilated left atrium. Left ventricular function severely impaired (ejection fraction 24 per cent).

QUESTIONS

1. What does this ECG show?
2. What is the mechanism of this?
3. What are the likely causes?
4. What are the key issues in managing this patient?

ECG ANALYSIS

Rate	72/min
Rhythm	Ventricular pacing
QRS axis	Left axis deviation (−48°)
P waves	Occasionally visible
PR interval	N/A
QRS duration	Prolonged (194 ms)
T waves	Abnormal
QTc interval	Prolonged (540 ms)

ANSWERS

1. There are occasional P waves visible between some (but not all) of the QRS complexes and occasional P waves can be seen deforming the ST segment. There is however no association between P waves and QRS complexes, indicating complete heart block. In addition, the QRS complexes are broad and preceded by a distinct 'spike' – this is **ventricular pacing**. The patient has had a VVI permanent pacemaker implanted for a diagnosis of complete heart block.

2. The 'spike' is an electrical discharge from a pacemaker, either temporary or permanent. In this case, a permanent single chamber or VVI (see coding schema below) pacemaker has been implanted to relieve symptoms of syncope. This paces the ventricle at a preset rate, in this case 72/min. If a ventricular depolarization is sensed, the pacemaker is 'inhibited' – all the beats on this ECG are 'paced' beats.

3. The pacemaker has been implanted because of complete heart block. The rate of the escape rhythm of the ventricles of approximately 15–40/min is inadequate for most activities and causes fatigue, dizziness and syncope.

4. The pacemaker to be implanted must be chosen with care. Insertion of a VVI pacemaker when there are P waves may cause symptoms due to 'pacemaker syndrome', when an atrial contraction against a closed tricuspid valve during systole may produce a wave of blood to flow retrogradely into the cerebral veins.

Generally speaking, in an active individual, physiological pacing with a 'dual chamber' or DDD pacemaker will harness atrial contractility and timing to optimize cardiac function.

COMMENTARY

- Pacemakers are described by pacing codes:
  - The first letter of the code identifies the chambers that can be paced (A – atrium, V – ventricle, D – dual)
  - The second letter of the code identifies the chambers that can be sensed (A – atrium, V – ventricle, D – dual)
  - The third letter of the code identifies what the pacemaker does if it detects intrinsic activity (I – inhibited, T – triggered, D – dual)
  - The fourth letter denotes whether rate-responsiveness (R) is present
  - The fifth letter identifies anti-tachycardia functions, if present (P – pacing, S – shock delivered, D – dual)
- The most commonly encountered pacemakers are:
  - VVI – a single lead pacemaker that senses ventricular activity; if no activity is detected, the pacemaker will take over cardiac rhythm by pacing the ventricle.
  - AAI – the pacemaker has a single lead, this time sensing atrial activity; if no activity is detected, the pacemaker paces the atrium.
  - DDD – there are pacemaker leads in both atrium and ventricle and so it senses activity in both chambers. It can pace atrium, ventricle or both sequentially.
- AAIR, VVIR and DDDR – are rate-responsive varieties of the above. The pacemaker adjusts its pacing rate according to the patient's level of activity to mimic physiological response to exercise. Several parameters can monitor activity, including vibration through a piezo-electric crystal, respiration and blood temperature.

Further reading

Making Sense of the ECG 4th edition: Pacemakers and implantable cardioverter defibrillators, p 209.

Epstein AE, DiMarco JP, Ellenbogen KA *et al.* ACC/AHA/ HRS 2008 guidelines for device-based therapy of cardiac rhythm abnormalities. A Report of the American College of Cardiology/American Heart Association task force on practice guidelines (writing committee to revise the ACC/AHA/NASPE 2002 guideline update for implantation of cardiac pacemakers and antiarrhythmia devices). *J Am Coll Cardiol* 2008; **51**: e1–62.

The Task Force on Cardiac Pacing and Resynchronization Therapy of the European Society of Cardiology (ESC). 2013 ESC guidelines on cardiac pacing and cardiac resynchronization therapy. *Eur Heart J* 2013; **34**: 2281–329.

CASE 37

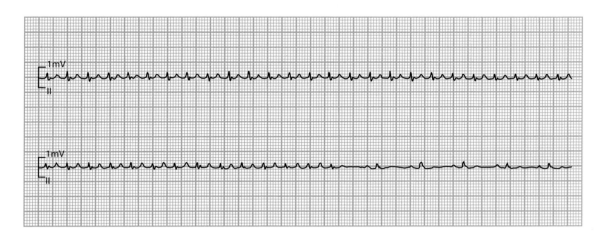

CLINICAL SCENARIO

Male, aged 22 years.

Presenting complaint
Rapid regular palpitations.

History of presenting complaint
Six-month history of episodic rapid regular palpitations. The current episode started suddenly 2 h prior to presentation.

Past medical history
Nil.

Examination
Pulse: 158/min, regular.
Blood pressure: 118/80.
JVP: normal.
Heart sounds: normal (tachycardic).
Chest auscultation: unremarkable.

Investigations
FBC: Hb 15.4, WCC 6.3, platelets 317.
U&E: Na 141, K 4.7, urea 4.8, creatinine 75.
Chest X-ray: normal heart size, clear lung fields.

QUESTIONS

1. What arrhythmia is seen in the initial part of this recording?
2. What intervention is likely to have been made at the point the rhythm changes?
3. What other interventions could have produced a similar result?

ECG ANALYSIS

Rate	158/min (during AVNRT)
Rhythm	Initially AVNRT, followed by sinus rhythm
QRS axis	Unable to assess (single lead)
P waves	Buried within QRS complexes during AVNRT (normal during sinus rhythm)
PR interval	Normal (180 ms) during sinus rhythm
QRS duration	Normal (100 ms) during AVNRT
T waves	Normal
QTc interval	Normal (438 ms) during sinus rhythm

ANSWERS

1. The first part of the recording shows a regular narrow complex tachycardia (158/min) with P waves buried within the QRS complexes (note the slight difference in shape of the QRS complexes during the tachycardia compared to those during sinus rhythm). This is **atrioventricular nodal re-entry tachycardia** (AVNRT). Other possibilities include:
   - atrioventricular re-entry tachycardia (AVRT), although in AVRT inverted P waves are often seen halfway between QRS complexes
   - atrial flutter with 2:1 atrioventricular block, although one would normally expect to see evidence of flutter waves.

2. The intervention performed is **carotid sinus massage**, which briefly blocks the atrioventricular node and terminates the arrhythmia. This rules out atrial flutter (carotid sinus massage would help reveal flutter waves but would not terminate atrial flutter).

3. Other interventions that can briefly block the atrioventricular node, terminating AVNRT, include the Valsalva manoeuvre or the administration of intravenous adenosine.

COMMENTARY

- The mechanism of AVNRT is discussed in Case 29.
- Vagal manoeuvres such as carotid sinus massage or the Valsalva manoeuvre are often effective in terminating episodes of AVNRT (and also AVRT).
- Applying an ice-filled glove to the face can also be effective, particularly in children who may struggle to perform a Valsalva manoeuvre.
- Do not use the old-fashioned vagal manoeuvre of applying eyeball pressure, as this can cause eyeball trauma.
- Do not use carotid sinus massage in individuals with known or suspected carotid or cerebrovascular disease, including those with carotid bruits.

Further reading

Making Sense of the ECG 4th edition: Atrioventricular nodal re-entry tachycardia, p 73.

Katritsis DG, Camm AJ. Atrioventricular nodal reentrant tachycardia. *Circulation* 2010; **122**: 831–40.

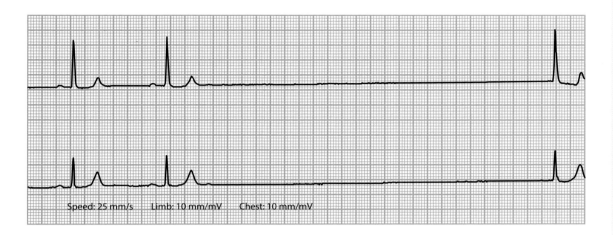

Speed: 25 mm/s   Limb: 10 mm/mV   Chest: 10 mm/mV

CLINICAL SCENARIO

Male, aged 69 years.

Presenting complaint
Felt unwell while driving.

History of presenting complaint
Occasional episodes of dizziness. One episode of collapse and unconsciousness while driving resulted in admission following a road traffic accident.

Past medical history
Nil of note.

Examination
Pulse: 45/min with long pauses.
Blood pressure: 124/78.
JVP: not elevated.
Heart sounds: normal.
Chest auscultation: unremarkable.
No peripheral oedema.

Investigations
FBC: Hb 13.9, WCC 6.6, platelets 203.
U&E: Na 139, K 3.9, urea 5.0, creatinine 109.
Chest X-ray: normal heart size, clear lung fields.
Echocardiogram: structurally normal valves, normal left ventricular function.

QUESTIONS

1. What does this ECG show?
2. What is the mechanism of this?
3. What are the key issues in managing this patient?

ECG ANALYSIS

Rate	45/min, followed by a 5.2 s pause
Rhythm	Sinus bradycardia followed by sinus arrest, then a junctional escape beat
QRS axis	Unable to assess
P waves	Normal (when present)
PR interval	Borderline prolonged (200 ms)
QRS duration	Normal (80 ms)
T waves	Normal
QTc interval	Normal (420 ms)

ANSWERS

1. This ECG rhythm strip shows two leads. There are two sinus beats, with a bradycardic heart rate of 45/min. There is then a pause of 5.2 s, during which no P waves are present. This is followed by a junctional escape beat. This is an episode of **sinus arrest**. The preceding sinus bradycardia is suggestive of underlying **sinus node dysfunction** (SND).

2. The sinus node fails to discharge reliably and 'on time' – there is cessation of P wave activity for a variable and unpredictable time period (compare this with sinoatrial block – Case 20). It can also be caused by excessive vagal inhibition, infarction, fibrosis, acute myocarditis, cardiomyopathy, drugs (digoxin, procainamide, quinidine) or amyloidosis. A slower subsidiary pacemaker further down the conduction pathway will sometimes take over – in this case, the atrioventricular junction (as evidenced by a beat with a narrow QRS complex but no preceding P wave).

3. If asymptomatic, no treatment is required, although drugs that can disrupt sinus node function should be withdrawn. Symptoms include sudden onset of confusion, breathlessness, syncope, chest pain, fatigue, or, if the event occurs at night, disturbed sleep. Symptoms can be relieved by implanting a permanent pacemaker. An atrial (AAI) pacemaker monitors and paces the atrium. Some patients also demonstrate atrioventricular conduction problems and a dual chamber (DDD) pacemaker is necessary to restore atrioventricular sequential pacing.

COMMENTARY

- Sinus arrest should be distinguished from sinoatrial block. In sinus arrest, the sinoatrial node stops firing for a variable time period, so the next P wave occurs after a *variable* interval. In sinoatrial block there is a pause with one or more absent P waves, and then the next P wave appears exactly where predicted – in other words, the sinoatrial node continues to 'keep time', but its impulses are not transmitted beyond the node to the atria.

- Sinus arrest and sinoatrial block can both be features of sick sinus syndrome. Other features of sick sinus syndrome can include sinus bradycardia (as seen here), brady-tachy syndrome and atrial fibrillation.

- Offer appropriate advice to patients who drive a vehicle and who suffer from presyncope or syncope – very often, they will be barred from driving until the problem has been diagnosed and/or corrected as appropriate. Driving regulations vary between countries. In the UK, information on the medical aspects of fitness to drive can be found on the website of the Driver and Vehicle Licensing Agency (www.dvla.gov.uk).

Further reading

Making Sense of the ECG 4th edition: Sinus bradycardia, p 54; Sinus arrest, p 94; P waves are intermittently absent, p 122.

CASE 39

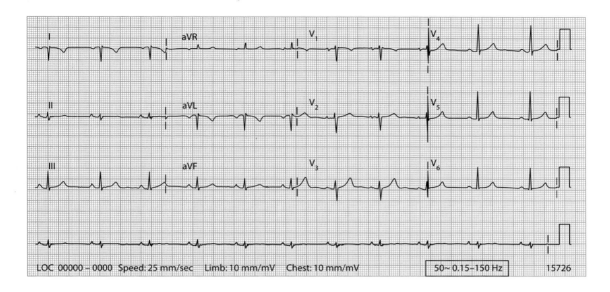

LOC 00000 – 0000   Speed: 25 mm/sec   Limb: 10 mm/mV   Chest: 10 mm/mV | 50~ 0.15–150 Hz | 15726

CLINICAL SCENARIO

Male, aged 24 years.

Presenting complaint
Routine ECG for insurance medical.

History of presenting complaint
No history – normally fit and well.

Past medical history
No prior medical history.

Examination
Pulse: 66/min, regular.
Blood pressure: 120/74.
JVP: not elevated.
Heart sounds: normal.
Chest auscultation: unremarkable.
No peripheral oedema.

Investigations
FBC: Hb 13.8, WCC 5.1, platelets 345.
U&E: Na 143, K 4.8, urea 4.7, creatinine 68.
Chest X-ray: normal heart size, clear lung fields.

QUESTIONS

1. What does this ECG show?
2. What is the cause of these ECG appearances?
3. What should you do next?

ECG ANALYSIS

Rate	66/min
Rhythm	Sinus rhythm
QRS axis	Right axis deviation (+152°)
P waves	Inverted in leads I and aVL, biphasic in lead aVR
PR interval	Normal (160 ms)
QRS duration	Normal (70 ms)
T waves	Inverted in leads I and aVL, upright in lead aVR
QTc interval	Normal (420 ms)

ANSWERS

1. This ECG has an unusual appearance:
   - There is extreme right axis deviation (+ 152°), and a positive QRS complex in lead aVR.
   - The QRS complexes in leads I and aVL are negative, and there is P wave and T wave inversion in these leads too.
2. These appearances are difficult to account for clinically – although similar appearances are seen in the limb leads in dextrocardia, we would also expect to find abnormalities in the chest leads in dextrocardia (whereas in this patient the chest leads are normal). Moreover, the patient's clinical examination and chest X-ray have not shown dextrocardia. This patient's ECG appearances are therefore due to **misplacement of the right and left arm electrodes**.
3. Check the ECG electrode positioning and reposition the right and left arm electrodes on the appropriate limb, so that the ECG can be repeated with all the electrodes in the correct place. When this patient's ECG was repeated, with the arm electrodes positioned correctly, it was found to be normal.

COMMENTARY

- It is thought that errors in electrode placement are made in up to 4 per cent of ECG recordings. When recording an ECG it is essential to check the electrode positioning carefully, as electrode misplacement can cause significant changes in the ECG's appearance and therefore lead to diagnosis (and treatment) errors.
- Any permutation of the limb and chest electrodes is theoretically possible, but the commonest electrode placement errors involve switching two of the limb electrodes or two of the chest electrodes.
- Always assess ECGs in the patient's clinical context, and ECG abnormalities that are unexpected or 'don't make sense' should always prompt a check of whether the ECG was recorded correctly.
- When an electrode placement error is recognized, repeat the ECG (with correct electrode placement) at the earliest opportunity.

Further reading

Making Sense of the ECG 4th edition: Performing an ECG recording, p 21; Electrode placement, p 23; Electrode misplacement, p 203.

Rudiger A, Hellermann JP, Mukherjee R *et al.* Electrocardiographic artifacts due to electrode misplacement and their frequency in different clinical settings. *Am J Emerg Med* 2007; **25**: 174–8.

The Society for Cardiological Science and Technology: Clinical Guidelines by Consensus. Recording a standard 12-lead electrocardiogram: an approved methodology. February 2010. Available for download from www.scst.org.uk.

CASE 40

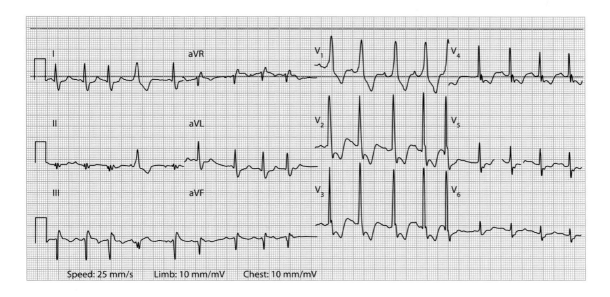

Speed: 25 mm/s   Limb: 10 mm/mV   Chest: 10 mm/mV

CLINICAL SCENARIO

Female, aged 81 years.

Presenting complaint
Severe central chest pain.

History of presenting complaint
Patient was walking to local shops. Experienced rapid onset of severe central crushing chest pain, associated with breathlessness and nausea. Similar to (but much worse than) her usual angina.

Past medical history
Exertional angina for many years.
Mild hypertension.
Type 2 diabetes mellitus.

Examination
Pulse: 108/min, regular with occasional ectopic beats.
Blood pressure: 108/76.
JVP: not elevated.
Heart sounds: normal.
Chest auscultation: unremarkable.
No peripheral oedema.

Investigations
FBC: Hb 12.1, WCC 4.7, platelets 390.
U&E: Na 141, K 4.9, urea 5.1, creatinine 143.
Troponin I: elevated at 457 (after 6 h).
Chest X-ray: mild cardiomegaly.
Echocardiogram: trace of mitral regurgitation but valve structurally normal. Left ventricle mildly impaired (ejection fraction 52 per cent), with posterior wall hypokinesia.

QUESTIONS

1. What does this ECG show?
2. What is the mechanism of this?
3. What treatment would be appropriate in this patient?

ECG ANALYSIS

Rate	108/min
Rhythm	Sinus rhythm with occasional ventricular ectopic beats
QRS axis	Left axis deviation (+36°)
P waves	Normal
PR interval	Normal (160 ms)
QRS duration	Upper limit of normal (120 ms)
T waves	Limb leads - normal.
	Chest leads - merged with ST segment.
QTc interval	Prolonged (480 ms)

Additional comments

There are tall dominant R waves in leads V1–V4 with ST segment depression.

ANSWERS

1. This ECG shows tall dominant R waves in leads with ST segment depression in the anterior chest leads. This is an **acute posterior ST segment elevation myocardial infarction (STEMI)**.
2. Posterior STEMI results from occlusion of the coronary artery supplying the posterior wall of the heart – in 70 per cent of cases, the right coronary artery (and in the remainder the circumflex artery).
3. Aspirin 300 mg orally (then 75 mg once daily), clopidogrel 300 mg orally (then 75 mg once daily), glyceryl trinitrate sublingually, pain relief (intravenous opiate plus an anti-emetic), oxygen if hypoxic. Prompt restoration of myocardial blood flow is required with primary percutaneous coronary intervention (PCI) or, if primary PCI is not available, thrombolysis.

COMMENTARY

- On a conventional ECG, the usual STEMI appearances of pathological Q waves, ST segment elevation and inverted T waves will, in a posterior STEMI, be seen as *reciprocal* changes in the anterior leads V1–V3, i.e. *R waves* (instead of Q waves), ST segment *depression* (instead of elevation) and *upright* T waves (rather than inverted) when viewed from leads V1–V3.
- The hallmark ST segment elevation of an acute STEMI is not seen in an acute posterior myocardial infarction unless an ECG is recorded using posterior leads, V7–V9, on the back of the chest. Posterior myocardial infarctions are therefore commonly overlooked, or misdiagnosed as anterior wall ischaemia. Using posterior leads helps to distinguish between the two diagnoses.
- In the clinical context of acute chest pain with ST segment depression in the anterior or anteroseptal leads, always consider the possibility of posterior myocardial infarction.
- Posterior myocardial infarction is one cause of a 'dominant' R wave in lead V1. Other causes are:
  - right ventricular hypertrophy
  - Wolff–Parkinson–White syndrome with a left-sided accessory pathway.

Further reading

Making Sense of the ECG 4th edition: Acute posterior myocardial infarction, p 174.

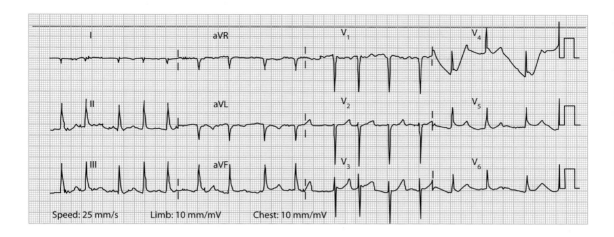

Speed: 25 mm/s   Limb: 10 mm/mV   Chest: 10 mm/mV

CLINICAL SCENARIO

Female, aged 83 years.

Presenting complaint
Found collapsed at home.

History of presenting complaint
Patient found lying on the floor of her home by a neighbour. She had slipped and fallen the previous evening when preparing to go to bed, and was found 11 h later having been on the floor all night. She had fractured her right hip and was unable to stand.

Past medical history
Stroke 4 years earlier (full recovery).

Examination
Reduced conscious level (Glasgow Coma Scale score 11/15).
Right leg shortened and externally rotated.
Temperature: 30.8°C.
Pulse: 96/min, irregularly irregular.
Blood pressure: 98/54.
JVP: not elevated.
Heart sounds: normal.
Chest auscultation: unremarkable.
No peripheral oedema.

Investigations
FBC: Hb 11.8, WCC 17.1, platelets 182.
U&E: Na 134, K 5.1, urea 11.7, creatinine 148.
Chest X-ray: normal heart size, clear lung fields.
Creatine kinase: elevated at 1565.

QUESTIONS

1. What does this ECG show?
2. What is the cause of these ECG appearances?
3. What other ECG findings may be seen in this condition?
4. What treatment is indicated?

ECG ANALYSIS

Rate	96/min
Rhythm	Atrial fibrillation
QRS axis	Right axis deviation (+98°)
P waves	Absent (atrial fibrillation)
PR interval	Not applicable
QRS duration	Normal (90 ms)
T waves	Normal
QTc interval	Prolonged (472 ms)

Additional comments

J waves (also known as 'Osborn waves') are visible in lead V4.

ANSWERS

1. This ECG shows atrial fibrillation with J waves, also known as Osborn waves. The J wave is a small positive deflection seen at the junction between the QRS complex and the ST segment and is usually best seen in the inferior limb leads and the lateral chest leads (in this case the J waves are most clearly seen in lead V4). The corrected QT interval is prolonged at 472 ms.
2. Hypothermia (the patient's temperature is 30.8°C).
3. J waves, atrial fibrillation and prolongation of the QT interval are all features of hypothermia. In addition, the ECG in hypothermia may also show broadening of the QRS complexes, lengthening of the PR interval, atrioventricular block, ventricular arrhythmias and asystole.
4. The treatment of hypothermia includes gradual rewarming and the administration, where appropriate, of warm intravenous fluids and warm humidified oxygen. Careful monitoring of vital signs and of the ECG is required. Passive rewarming is suitable for most patients with mild hypothermia; consider active rewarming for those with moderate or severe hypothermia. Manage co-morbidities (e.g. sepsis or, in this case, a hip fracture) as appropriate.

COMMENTARY

- J waves, also known as Osborn waves, are characterized by a dome- or hump-shaped deflection of the ECG at the junction of the QRS complex and the ST segment (the J point). J waves have been reported to be present in around 80 per cent of ECGs in hypothermic patients (below 33°C), but they are also sometimes seen in patients with a normal body temperature and are therefore not completely specific for hypothermia.
- A variety of arrhythmias can be seen in hypothermia. Sinus tachycardia is the earliest abnormality, followed (as core temperature falls) by sinus bradycardia, then atrial ectopics and atrial fibrillation (often with a slow ventricular rate). As the temperature falls further, the QRS complexes become increasingly broad and the risk of ventricular fibrillation increases. Finally, asystole occurs.
- Ventricular fibrillation can be refractory to defibrillation in the severely hypothermic patient. In patients with a core temperature below 30°C, the onset of ventricular tachycardia or fibrillation should be treated with an attempt at defibrillation – if this is ineffective, defer further attempts until the patient's core temperature is above 30°C.

Further reading

Making Sense of the ECG 4th edition: Are J waves present? p 176.

Epstein E, Anna K. Accidental hypothermia. *BMJ* 2006; **332**: 706–9.

Mattu A, Brady W, Perron A. Electrocardiographic manifestations of hypothermia. *Am J Emerg Med* 2002; **20**: 314–26.

CASE 42

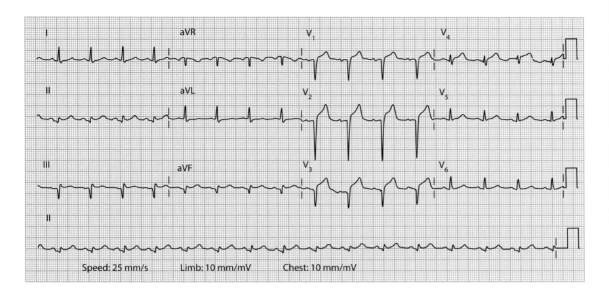

Speed: 25 mm/s   Limb: 10 mm/mV   Chest: 10 mm/mV

CLINICAL SCENARIO

Male, aged 65 years.

Presenting complaint
Breathlessness on exertion, but no chest pain.

History of presenting complaint
Patient had a heart attack 6 months previously. Never returned to previous activity levels. In past few weeks, noticed more breathlessness than usual – had to avoid stairs as much as possible, and steep paths were now impossible. Occasional paroxysmal nocturnal dyspnoea. Patient had a similar ECG in his wallet, given to him on discharge from previous admission.

Past medical history
No history of lung disease.

Examination
Pulse: 96/min, regular.
Blood pressure: 114/66.
JVP: not elevated.
Heart sounds: normal.
Chest auscultation: bilateral inspiratory crackles.
No peripheral oedema.

Investigations
FBC: Hb 12.7, WCC 8.0, platelets 284.
U&E: Na 139, K 4.6, urea 4.8, creatinine 124.
Troponin I: negative.
Chest X-ray: enlarged left ventricle. Pulmonary oedema.

QUESTIONS

1. What does this ECG show?
2. What would be the most useful investigation?
3. What are the key issues in managing this patient?

ECG ANALYSIS

Rate	96/min
Rhythm	Sinus rhythm
QRS axis	Normal (−10°)
P waves	Normal
PR interval	Normal (160 ms)
QRS duration	Normal (100 ms)
T waves	Normal
QTc interval	Mildly prolonged (455 ms)

Additional comments

There are deep anterior Q waves with persistent ST segment elevation.

ANSWERS

1. Deep Q waves with persistent ST segment elevation in leads V1–V4, 6 months after a previous myocardial infarction, is suggestive of a **left ventricular aneurysm**.
2. An echocardiogram would confirm the presence of a left ventricular aneurysm and allow assessment of left ventricular function and any valvular dysfunction. A cardiac magnetic resonance scan is also useful for delineating the extent of any aneurysmal segment and also assessing myocardial viability.
3. Although the ST segment elevation on the admission ECG may suggest a new infarction, the history (progressive breathlessness without chest pain) is not compatible with this diagnosis. A chest X-ray will show an abnormal silhouette and the troponin level will be in the normal range. Comparison with a pre-discharge ECG from the time of his previous infarction allows confirmation that the ST segment elevation is

longstanding. Patients may present with heart failure, an embolic event, intractable arrhythmias or chest pain. Treatment of heart failure, rhythm abnormalities and anticoagulation are required as appropriate. Surgical resection of the aneurysm (aneurysmectomy) may improve symptoms.

COMMENTARY

- Coronary artery disease and acute myocardial infarction are the most common causes of a left ventricular aneurysm. Rarer causes include trauma, Chagas' disease and sarcoidosis.
- Left ventricular aneurysm is a late complication of myocardial infarction, seen in around 10 per cent of survivors.
- Left ventricular aneurysm may present as:
  - breathlessness – aneurysmal tissue is non-contractile, so an extensive aneurysm may cause loss of a large proportion of left ventricular function and lead to symptoms and signs of heart failure
  - ventricular arrhythmia – the ischaemic border zone is a substrate for ventricular ectopic beats and ventricular tachycardia
  - sudden death – due to ventricular arrhythmias, or to spontaneous rupture of the aneurysmal segment
  - chest pain – the border zone between infarcted aneurysmal tissue and healthy, non-infarcted myocardium can become ischaemic
  - embolism – thrombus may form in a ventricular aneurysm, due to relative stasis of blood, and embolize.

Further reading

Making Sense of the ECG 4th edition: Are the ST segments elevated? p 159; Left ventricular aneurysm, p 165.

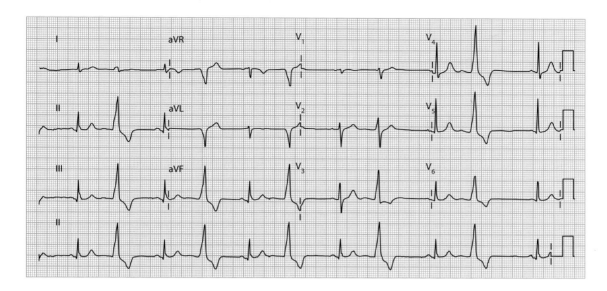

CLINICAL SCENARIO

Male, aged 78 years.

Presenting complaint
Asymptomatic.

History of presenting complaint
Patient attended for preoperative screening for a right inguinal hernia repair. His pulse was noted to be irregular, and this ECG was performed.

Past medical history
Right inguinal hernia. No prior cardiovascular history.

Examination
Pulse: 66/min, regularly irregular.
Blood pressure: 134/76.
JVP: not elevated.
Heart sounds: regularly irregular.
Chest auscultation: unremarkable.
No peripheral oedema.

Investigations
FBC: Hb 13.5, WCC 6.1, platelets 318.
U&E: Na 137, K 4.2, urea 4.8, creatinine 80.
Thyroid function: normal.
Chest X-ray: normal heart size, clear lung fields.
Echocardiogram: normal cardiac structure and function.

QUESTIONS

1. What arrhythmia does this ECG show?
2. Where in the heart has this arrhythmia originated?

ECG ANALYSIS

Rate	66/min
Rhythm	Ventricular bigeminy
QRS axis	Normal (+80°) for sinus beats, inferior axis for ventricular ectopic beats
P waves	Present for sinus beats
PR interval	160 ms
QRS duration	Normal (80 ms) for sinus beats, broad (140 ms) for ventricular ectopic beats
T waves	Normal for sinus beats, inverted for ventricular ectopic beats
QTc interval	Normal (440 ms)

ANSWERS

1. In this ECG every normal sinus beat is followed by a broad and abnormally shaped QRS complex, a ventricular ectopic beat (VEB). This 1:1 coupling between sinus beats and VEBs is called **ventricular bigeminy**.
2. As the name suggests, VEBs arise within the ventricles. In this case the VEBs have a left bundle branch block morphology in the chest leads, indicating an origin in the right ventricle. The VEBs also have an inferior axis in the limb leads (positive complexes in leads II, III and aVF) indicating an origin in the basal part of the ventricle. Taken together, these features suggest the most likely origin of the VEBs is in the basal right ventricle, most probably the right ventricular outflow tract.

COMMENTARY

- An ectopic beat arises earlier than the next normal (sinus) beat would have occurred (in contrast to escape beats, which arise later than expected).

- VEBs cause broad QRS complexes (unlike supraventricular ectopics, which usually cause narrow QRS complexes). The VEB, having arisen within the ventricular myocardium, has to conduct from myocyte to myocyte in order to depolarize the ventricles – this is slower than conduction via the His–Purkinje system, and hence ventricular depolarization takes longer than it would with a normal sinus beat.
- VEBs arising from the right ventricle have a left bundle branch block morphology, and those arising from the left ventricle have a right bundle branch block morphology.
- On checking the radial pulse of a patient with bigeminy, the VEBs usually feel weaker than the normal sinus beats (because the ventricle has not filled fully by the time systole occurs). As a result, VEBs may sometimes be missed on palpation of the radial pulse. Patients with ventricular bigeminy are therefore sometimes mistakenly diagnosed as being bradycardic when their pulse is taken at the wrist, if only the sinus beats are counted. Even automated monitoring equipment (e.g. blood pressure monitors, pulse oximeters) can sometimes underestimate the heart rate by 'missing' the VEBs. Careful inspection of an ECG will reveal the correct heart rate.
- The normal sinus beat after the VEB can also feel stronger than usual, as there will have been a slightly longer period for ventricular filling due to the compensatory pause after the VEB ('extrasystolic potentiation').
- For more information on the investigation and management of VEBs, see the commentary on Case 9.

Further reading

Making Sense of the ECG 4th edition: Ventricular ectopic beats, p 79.

Ng GA. Treating patients with ventricular ectopic beats. *Heart* 2006; **92**: 1707–12.

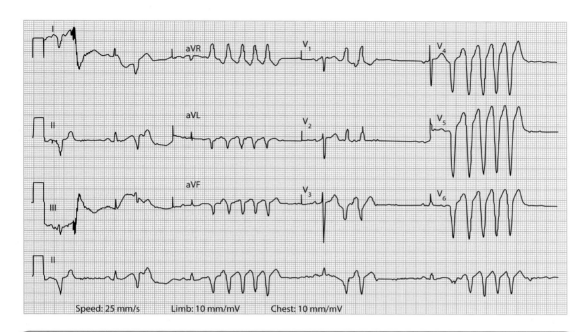

Speed: 25 mm/s   Limb: 10 mm/mV   Chest: 10 mm/mV

CLINICAL SCENARIO

Male, aged 26 years.

Presenting complaint
Breathlessness. Persistent nocturnal cough. Dizziness.

History of presenting complaint
Had been fit and well until 2 months ago when he had a viral infection. Never really regained fitness afterwards. Had had several courses of antibiotics from family doctor but his symptoms persisted. Frequent nocturnal waking with breathlessness. Became worried when he found he was breathless walking around his flat and he noticed his pulse was very erratic.

Past medical history
Nil else of note.
Smokes 10 cigarettes per day.
Drinks 12 units alcohol per week.

No family history of heart disease.

Examination
Pulse: 108/min, irregular.
Blood pressure: 118/88.
JVP: elevated by 4 cm.
Heart sounds: normal.
Chest auscultation: bi-basal crackles.
Pitting peripheral oedema to mid-calf.

Investigations
FBC: Hb 12.2, WCC 8.1, platelets 346.
U&E: Na 136, K 4.9, urea 7.8, creatinine 124.
Thyroid function: normal.
Troponin I: negative.
Chest X-ray: enlarged left ventricle. Pulmonary oedema.
Echocardiogram: Dilated left ventricle with poor function. Mildly impaired right ventricular function. Functional mitral regurgitation.

QUESTIONS

1. What does this ECG show?
2. What is the likely cause?
3. What are the key issues in managing this patient?

ECG ANALYSIS

Rate	108/min overall, but very variable
Rhythm	Underlying sinus rhythm with frequent bursts of non-sustained ventricular tachycardia
QRS axis	Normal (+45°) in sinus rhythm, extreme axis deviation in VT
P waves	Normal
PR interval	Normal (172 ms)
QRS duration	Normal (90 ms) in sinus rhythm, broad complexes in ventricular tachycardia
T waves	Normal morphology where seen
QTc interval	Difficult to assess

ANSWERS

1. Underlying sinus rhythm is seen with normal axis. There are frequent runs of non-sustained broad complex tachycardia with a marked change in axis. These are bursts of **ventricular tachycardia (VT)**.

2. The underlying diagnosis is most likely to be a dilated cardiomyopathy secondary to viral myocarditis.

3. Treatment is aimed at controlling the signs and symptoms of congestive cardiac failure until resolution occurs – this may take weeks or months (if at all). Patients usually respond to a combination of loop diuretic, angiotensin-converting enzyme (ACE) inhibitor (titrated to the maximum tolerated dose while monitoring renal function), and beta blocker (in escalating dose). Failure to respond to treatment warrants full investigation. Antiarrhythmic drugs may be needed for ventricular tachyarrhythmias, and an implantable cardioverter defibrillator (ICD) may be required for patients at high risk of cardiac arrest. Surgical options include a left ventricular assist device (LVAD) to support the function of the failing heart, and cardiac transplantation for those with severe heart failure that fails to improve.

COMMENTARY

- Broad-complex tachycardia is due to VT, or to supraventricular tachycardia (SVT) with aberrant conduction (such as bundle branch block or ventricular pre-excitation). Where there is doubt about the diagnosis, it should be assumed to be VT until proven otherwise.

- Most cases (80%) of broad complex tachycardia are due to VT, and the likelihood of VT (rather than SVT with aberrant conduction) is even higher when structural heart disease is present. Haemodynamic stability is not a reliable guide in distinguishing between VT and SVT with aberrant conduction, as VT can be remarkably well tolerated by some patients.

- A very reliable ECG indicator of VT is the presence of **atrioventricular dissociation**, where the atria and ventricles are seen to be working independently. Atrioventricular dissociation is indicated by:
  - independent P wave activity
  - fusion beats
  - capture beats.

- Other ECG features can also provide clues to the diagnosis. Most patients with SVT and aberrant conduction will have a QRS complex morphology that looks like a typical LBBB or RBBB pattern. Patients with VT will often (but not always) have more unusual-looking QRS complexes which don't fit a typical bundle branch block pattern.

- Many other ECG features suggest (but do not prove) a diagnosis of VT rather than SVT with aberrant conduction, including:
  - very broad QRS complexes (>160 ms)
  - extreme QRS axis deviation
  - concordance (same QRS direction) in leads V1–V6
  - an interval >100 ms from the start of the R wave to the deepest point of the S wave (this is called Brugada's sign) in one chest lead
  - a notch in the downstroke of the S wave (this is called Josephson's sign).

Further reading

Making Sense of the ECG 4th edition: Ventricular tachycardia, p 83; How do I distinguish between VT and SVT? p 86.

Alzand BSN, Crijns HJGM. Diagnostic criteria of broad QRS complex tachycardia: decades of evolution. *Europace* 2011; **13**: 465–72.

Jastrzebski M, Kukla P, Czarnecka D *et al.* Comparison of five electrocardiographic methods for differentiation of wide QRS-complex tachycardias. *Europace* 2012; **14**: 1165–71.

CASE 45

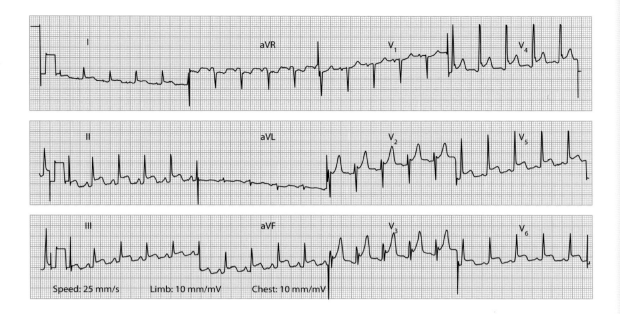

I   aVR   V₁   V₄

II   aVL   V₂   V₅

III   aVF   V₃   V₆

Speed: 25 mm/s   Limb: 10 mm/mV   Chest: 10 mm/mV

CLINICAL SCENARIO

Male, aged 25 years.

Presenting complaint
Central chest pain, exacerbated by lying supine and on deep inspiration.

History of presenting complaint
Viral symptoms for 1 week, with chest pain for 3 days.

Past medical history
Nil.

Examination
Patient in discomfort and sitting upright.
Temperature: 38.1°C.

Pulse: 110/min, regular.
Blood pressure: 128/80.
JVP: not elevated.
Heart sounds: soft pericardial friction rub.
Chest auscultation: unremarkable.
No peripheral oedema.

Investigations
FBC: Hb 15.2, WCC 9.2, platelets 364.
U&E: Na 141, K 4.4, urea 3.8, creatinine 58.
ESR and CRP: elevated.
Thyroid function: normal.
Chest X-ray: normal heart size, clear lung fields.

QUESTIONS

1. What does this ECG show?
2. What other tests would be appropriate?
3. What can cause this condition?
4. What are the treatment options?

ECG ANALYSIS

Rate	110/min
Rhythm	Sinus rhythm
QRS axis	Normal (+65°)
P waves	Normal
PR interval	Normal (160 ms)
QRS duration	Normal (80 ms)
T waves	Normal
QTc interval	Normal (433 ms)

Additional comments

There is widespread ST segment elevation (concave upward or 'saddle-shaped') in leads I, II, III, aVF and V2–V6, with reciprocal ST segment depression in lead aVR.

ANSWERS

1. This ECG shows widespread ST segment eleva-tion (concave upward or 'saddle-shaped') in leads I, II, III, aVF and V2–V6, with reciprocal ST segment depression in lead aVR. In the clini-cal context, these findings are consistent with a diagnosis of **pericarditis**.
2. In addition to those listed, other appropriate tests would include:
   - cardiac markers (troponin)
   - echocardiography
   - viral serology with or without other microbi-ology as indicated
   - autoantibody screen, complement levels, immunoglobulins.
3. Pericarditis has many causes, including:
   - idiopathic
   - infective (viral, bacterial, tuberculous, fun-gal, parasitic)
   - myocardial infarction (first few days)
   - Dressler's syndrome (1 month or more post-myocardial infarction)
   - uraemia
   - malignancy
   - connective tissue disease
   - radiotherapy
   - traumatic
   - drug-induced.
4. Direct treatment of the underlying cause is important where applicable. Anti-inflammatory drugs (e.g. aspirin, indometacin) can be effec-tive. Steroids can be considered in selected cases, but their use is controversial and so seek specialist advice. Colchicine can be useful in the management of relapsing pericarditis.

COMMENTARY

- The ST segment elevation of pericarditis is typi-cally widespread, appearing in more leads than one would normally expect for an acute myocar-dial infarction. The morphology of the ST seg-ment elevation is described as concave upwards or 'saddle shaped'. As the pericarditis settles, the ST segments gradually return to baseline and, in the longer term, there may be residual T wave inversion.
- Pericarditis can also cause depression of the PR segment, which is thought to be caused by atrial involvement in the inflammatory process. PR segment depression is a specific ECG feature of pericarditis and may be seen in any leads except aVR and V1 (where there may be PR segment elevation).
- Patients with pericarditis and ST segment eleva-tion will often have an elevation in their car-diac markers (troponin) as a result of a degree of coexistent myocarditis. It is important not to misdiagnose acute myocardial infarction, and a coronary angiogram may be required to clarify the diagnosis.
- Echocardiography is important to monitor for the appearance of a pericardial effusion (not always present, but may develop as a complica-tion). This can cause cardiac tamponade.
- The differential diagnosis of ST segment elevation includes acute myocardial infarction, left ventricular aneurysm, Prinzmetal's (vaso-spastic) angina, pericarditis, high take-off, left bundle branch block and Brugada syndrome.

Further reading

Making Sense of the ECG 4th edition: Are the ST segments elevated? p 159; Pericarditis, p 168; Is the PR segment elevated or depressed? p 135.

Marinella MA. Electrocardiographic manifestations and differential diagnosis of acute pericarditis. *Am Fam Physician* 1998; **57**: 699-704.

Oakley CM. Myocarditis, pericarditis and other pericardial diseases. *Heart* 2000; **84**: 449–54.

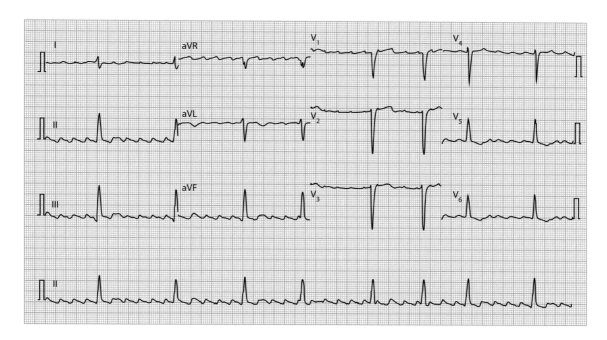

CLINICAL SCENARIO

Male, aged 73 years.

Presenting complaint
Exertional breathlessness.

History of presenting complaint
Six week history of exertional breathlessness. Also aware of an irregular heartbeat.

Past medical history
Hypertension.

Examination
Pulse: 51/min, irregular.

Blood pressure: 168/102.
JVP: not elevated.
Heart sounds: normal (but irregular rhythm).
Chest auscultation: bibasal inspiratory crackles.
Mild peripheral oedema.

Investigations
FBC: Hb 13.9, WCC 6.0, platelets 188.
U&E: Na 139, K 4.8, urea 9.4, creatinine 147.
Thyroid function: normal.
Chest X-ray: normal heart size, mild pulmonary congestion.
Echocardiogram: normal valves. Mild left ventricular hypertrophy with mildly impaired systolic function (ejection fraction 48 per cent).

QUESTIONS

1. What rhythm does this ECG show?
2. What are the key issues in managing this patient?

ECG ANALYSIS

Rate	51/min
Rhythm	Atrial flutter
QRS axis	Normal (+90°)
P waves	Not visible (flutter waves are present)
PR interval	N/A
QRS duration	Normal (112 ms)
T waves	Inverted in leads I, aVL, V5, V6
QTc interval	Normal (318 ms)

ANSWERS

1. There are low amplitude flutter waves at around 300/min which give a 'sawtooth' baseline: this is **atrial flutter**. There is *variable* atrioventricular block, giving rise to an irregularly irregular rhythm with a ventricular rate of around 51/min.

2. There are four key aspects to the treatment of atrial flutter:
   - Ventricular rate control – in this case, there is a high (and variable) degree of atrioventricular block and so the ventricular rate is relatively slow. Rate-controlling medication is therefore not required in this case, unless there is a marked increase in atrioventricular conduction (and therefore in ventricular rate) on exertion.
   - There is a thromboembolic risk in atrial flutter, and so consider the patient for antithrombotic therapy in the same way as for atrial fibrillation.
   - Electrical cardioversion can be very effective in restoring sinus rhythm and, as a general rule, atrial flutter is easier to cardiovert than atrial fibrillation.
   - Electrophysiological intervention with radiofrequency ablation of the atrial flutter re-entry circuit is an effective procedure with a success rate >95 per cent.

COMMENTARY

- Atrial flutter is indicated by the presence of a 'sawtooth' pattern of atrial activity with an atrial rate of approximately 300/min.
- Atrioventricular block can be variable in atrial flutter, and so the ventricular rhythm can be irregular. In such cases, the rhythm can be mistaken for atrial fibrillation.
- Rate controlling medication is not always necessary in atrial flutter (or in atrial fibrillation), as some cases have a normal (or even a slow) ventricular rate. However, assessing ventricular rate only at rest can underestimate how much the rate rises during periods of activity. It is therefore a good idea to assess ventricular rate not just at rest but also after a short period of exertion.

Further reading

Making Sense of the ECG 4th edition: Atrial flutter, p 64.
Waldo AL. Treatment of atrial flutter. *Heart* 2000; **84**: 227–32.

CASE 47

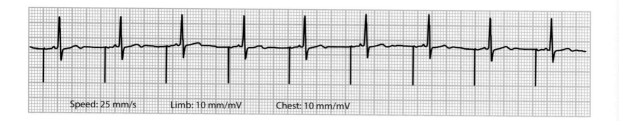

Speed: 25 mm/s   Limb: 10 mm/mV   Chest: 10 mm/mV

CLINICAL SCENARIO

Female, aged 63 years.

Presenting complaint
Asymptomatic – routine ECG performed at follow-up visit to cardiology outpatient clinic.

History of presenting complaint
Nil – patient currently asymptomatic.

Past medical history
Treated for sick sinus syndrome 2 years ago.

Examination
Pulse: 70/min, regular.
Blood pressure: 138/78.
JVP: not elevated.
Heart sounds: normal.
Chest auscultation: unremarkable.
No peripheral oedema.

Investigations
FBC: Hb 13.8, WCC 5.7, platelets 240.
U&E: Na 141, K 4.3, urea 2.8, creatinine 68.

QUESTIONS

1. What does this ECG show?
2. What device did this patient receive 2 years ago to treat their sick sinus syndrome?
3. Does this device have one electrode or two? How might you find out?
4. What do you understand by the term AAIR?

ECG ANALYSIS

Rate	70/min
Rhythm	Atrial pacing
QRS axis	–
P waves	Present following atrial pacing spike
PR interval	Short
QRS duration	Normal (80 ms)
T waves	Biphasic (initially positive but with negative terminal deflection)
QTc interval	Normal (350 ms)

Additional comments

Pacing spikes are evident prior to each P wave.

ANSWERS

1. There are sharp downward vertical deflections prior to each P wave. These represent pacing spikes. The position of these prior to the P wave indicates atrial pacing.
2. The patient has had a pacemaker implanted two years ago to treat their sick sinus syndrome.
3. It is not possible to say. The pacemaker is certainly capable of pacing the atria, as evidenced by pacing spikes followed by P waves, and an atrial pacing electrode must therefore be present. However, the absence of ventricular pacing does not rule out the possibility that a ventricular electrode is also present – if it is a dual chamber pacemaker, the ventricular lead may simply be monitoring ventricular activity but not supplying any pacing spikes at present. If in doubt, most patients with pacemakers will carry a pacemaker identity card. Failing that, a chest X-ray will reveal the number of pacing electrodes. This patient actually had a single chamber pacemaker (AAIR).
4. The term AAIR is a pacing code, and describes a pacemaker that paces the atrium, senses the atrium, is inhibited by intrinsic atrial activity, and is rate-responsive.

COMMENTARY

- Permanent pacemakers can be single chamber (a single electrode pacing/sensing either the right atrium or the right ventricle) or dual chamber (two electrodes, one to pace/sense the right atrium and another to pace/sense the right ventricle).
- For sick sinus syndrome, a single chamber atrial pacemaker is usually appropriate unless there are any problems (or potential problems) with atrioventricular node conduction, in which case a dual chamber pacemaker is a better option.
- Pacemakers can be identified on the ECG by their pacing spikes. The presence of a pacing spike followed by a P wave indicates atrial pacing. A pacing spike followed by a QRS complex indicates ventricular pacing.
- Pacemakers are described by pacing codes:
  - The first letter of the code identifies the chambers that can be paced (A – atrium, V – ventricle, D – dual).
  - The second letter of the code identifies the chambers that can be sensed (A – atrium, V – ventricle, D – dual).
  - The third letter of the code identifies what the pacemaker does if it detects intrinsic activity (I – inhibited, T – triggered, D – dual).
  - The fourth letter denotes whether rate-responsiveness (R) is present.
  - The fifth letter identifies anti-tachycardia functions, if present (P – pacing, S – shock delivered, D – dual).

Thus an AAIR pacemaker can pace the atrium. However, if it senses intrinsic atrial activity (normal P waves), it will be inhibited and stop pacing. The R indicates that it is rate-responsive, and can therefore increase its pacing rate (and thus the patient's heart rate) if it detects that the patient is undertaking physical exertion. Pacemakers can detect physical activity by monitoring a variety of indicators including vibration, respiration or blood temperature.

Further reading

Making Sense of the ECG 4th edition: Sick sinus syndrome, p 57; Pacemakers and implantable cardioverter defibrillators, p 209.

Morgan JM. Basics of cardiac pacing: selection and mode choice. *Heart* 2006 **92**: 850–54.

The Task Force on Cardiac Pacing and Resynchronization Therapy of the European Society of Cardiology (ESC). 2013 ESC guidelines on cardiac pacing and cardiac resynchronization therapy. *Eur Heart J* 2013; **34**: 2281–329.

CASE 48

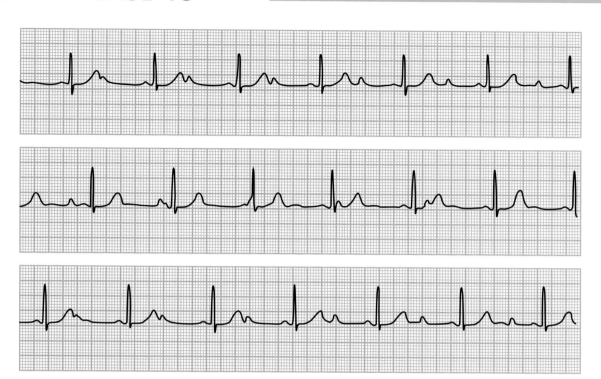

CLINICAL SCENARIO

Male, aged 71 years.

Presenting complaint
Asymptomatic.

History of presenting complaint
Asymptomatic (routine ECG performed for hypertension assessment).

Past medical history
Hypertension.

Examination
Pulse: 54/min, regular.
Blood pressure: 154/84.
JVP: cannon waves visible.
Heart sounds: normal.
Chest auscultation: unremarkable.
No peripheral oedema.

Investigations
FBC: Hb 14.3, WCC 6.6, platelets 344.
U&E: Na 140, K 3.9, urea 6.6, creatinine 105.
Thyroid function: normal.

QUESTIONS

1. What does this ECG show?
2. What is the mechanism of this?

ECG ANALYSIS

Rate	Atrial - 104/min
	Ventricular - 54/min
Rhythm	Sinus rhythm with atrial parasystole
QRS axis	Unable to assess (rhythm strip)
P waves	Two morphologies – normal and abnormal
PR interval	There is a normal PR interval for the 'sinus rhythm' P waves. The atrial parasystole P waves are non-conducted and so these do not have a PR interval.
QRS duration	Normal (80 ms)
T waves	Normal
QTc interval	Normal (399 ms)

ANSWERS

1. This ECG shows **atrial parasystole**.
2. Atrial parasystole occurs when there is a secondary pacemaker within the atria that fires in parallel with the sinoatrial node. Thus there are two simultaneous atrial rhythms – normal sinus rhythm (seen here at 54/min) in which each P wave is followed by a QRS complex, and a separate parasystolic rhythm (at a rate of 50/min) with P waves that are taller than the normal P waves. Because the two rates are slightly different, the parasystolic P waves can be seen to gradually 'march through' the normal sinus rhythm P waves.

COMMENTARY

- Parasystole is very rare. It can occur in the atria (atrial parasystole) or in the ventricles (ventricular parasystole). Ventricular parasystole is commoner.
- The ectopic focus in parasystole is surrounded by a region of myocardium that causes 'entrance block', protecting the ectopic focus from being depolarized by the normal beats. The ectopic focus is therefore able to function independently of the underlying rhythm.
- Parasystole can be continuous or intermittent.
- Occasional fusion beats (between an normal beat and a parasystolic beat) may be seen.

Further reading

Friedberg HD, Schamroth L. Atrial parasystole. *Br Heart J* 1970; **32**: 172–80.

CASE 49

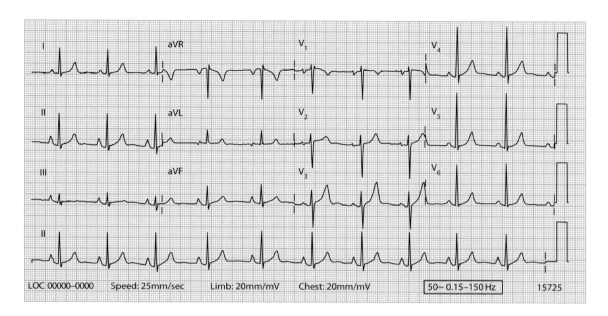

LOC 00000–0000   Speed: 25mm/sec   Limb: 20mm/mV   Chest: 20mm/mV   50~ 0.15–150 Hz   15725

CLINICAL SCENARIO

Male, aged 40 years.

Presenting complaint

Hypertension.

History of presenting complaint

Patient noted to be hypertensive (152/94) during routine check-up. This ECG was performed as part of his cardiovascular assessment.

Past medical history

Recently diagnosed hypertension – not on medication.

Examination

Pulse: 64/min, regular.
Blood pressure: 152/94.
JVP: not elevated.
Heart sounds: normal.
Chest auscultation: unremarkable.
No peripheral oedema.

Investigations

FBC: Hb 15.3, WCC 6.1, platelets 409.
U&E: Na 141, K 4.3, urea 5.9, creatinine 83.
Chest X-ray: normal heart size, clear lung fields.

QUESTIONS

1. What does this ECG show?
2. What would you do next?

ECG ANALYSIS

Rate	64/min
Rhythm	Sinus rhythm
QRS axis	Normal (+32°)
P waves	Normal
PR interval	Normal (160 ms)
QRS duration	Normal (70 ms)
T waves	Normal
QTc interval	Normal (430 ms)

Additional comments

The voltage calibration setting is 20 mm/mV, double the 'standard' setting.

ANSWERS

1. At first glance, this ECG might appear to meet a number of the diagnostic criteria for left ventricular hypertrophy (see Case 35). However, on closer inspection it can be seen that the voltage calibration has been set at 20mm/mV, which is double the standard setting (10 mm/mV). Therefore all the waves/complexes on the ECG will be twice their 'usual' size. When this is taken into account, the ECG is in fact **normal**.

2. Repeat the ECG at the standard calibration setting of 10 mm/mV (unless a different non-standard setting is required for a particular purpose).

COMMENTARY

- ECGs are normally recorded at a standard calibration setting of 10 mm/mV. In other words, a voltage of 1mV will cause a 10 mm deflection in the ECG tracing.
- The calibration setting is usually indicated on the ECG by an annotation (in this case 'Limb: 20 mm/mV Chest: 20 mm/mV' along the bottom of the ECG), and/or by a calibration marker (the upright 'box' at the far right of this recording, which shows what deflection is made by a voltage of 1mV). It is good practice to check the calibration settings on every ECG you examine.
- Many ECG machines will allow the calibration of the limb leads and the chest leads to be set independently.
- For the vast majority of ECGs, a standard setting of 10 mm/mV is appropriate. For patients with very large QRS complexes (e.g. as seen in left ventricular hypertrophy), sometimes at the standard setting the QRS complexes on adjacent lines can overlap and make interpretation difficult. Under these circumstances, a calibration of 5 mm/mV will halve the size of the complexes and may make the ECG easier to interpret. The use of double the normal calibration (20 mm/mV) is very unusual.

Further reading

Making Sense of the ECG 4th edition: Performing an ECG recording p 21; Incorrect calibration, p 204.

The Society for Cardiological Science and Technology: Clinical Guidelines by Consensus. Recording a standard 12-lead electrocardiogram: an approved methodology. February 2010. Available for download from www.scst.org.uk

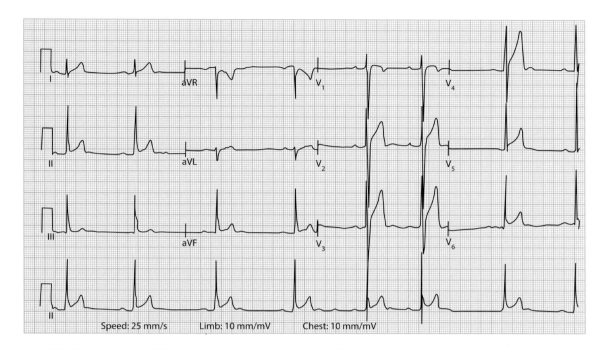

Speed: 25 mm/s   Limb: 10 mm/mV   Chest: 10 mm/mV

CLINICAL SCENARIO

Male, aged 29 years.

Presenting complaint
Chest pain.

History of presenting complaint
Usually fit and well. Patient was at a party with friends and had consumed quite a lot of alcohol – more than he usually drank. Friends reported that he then developed severe central chest pain which got progressively worse. They were concerned so called for an ambulance. Admitted to coronary care unit with a suspected acute myocardial infarction.

Past medical history
Nil of note.
Heavy smoker.

Examination
Pulse: 48/min, some variation with respiration.
Blood pressure: 148/96.
JVP: not elevated.
Heart sounds: normal.
Chest auscultation: unremarkable.
No peripheral oedema.

Investigations
FBC: Hb 13.9, WCC 8.1, platelets 233.
U&E: Na 137, K 4.2, urea 5.3, creatinine 88.
Troponin I: negative.
Chest X-ray: normal heart size, clear lung fields.
Echocardiogram: normal valves. Left ventricular function good (ejection fraction 67 per cent).

QUESTIONS

1. What does this ECG show?
2. What is the mechanism of this?
3. What are the likely causes?
4. What are the key issues in managing this patient?

ECG ANALYSIS

Rate	48/min
Rhythm	Sinus rhythm (with a degree of sinus arrhythmia)
QRS axis	Normal (+74°)
P waves	Normal
PR interval	Prolonged (232 ms)
QRS duration	Normal (114 ms)
T waves	Tall in V2–V4 ('hyperacute')
QTc interval	Normal (351 ms)

Additional comments

There is ST segment elevation in leads V2–V6.

ANSWERS

1. ST segment elevation most marked in the anterior chest leads. If these changes resolve as the chest pain resolves, and there is no subsequent troponin rise, this is consistent with myocardial ischaemia due to **coronary artery vasospasm** ('Prinzmetal's angina').

2. Coronary artery vasospasm leads to a reduction in blood supply to the myocardium supplied by the affected artery. ECG changes are not confined to the ST segment – hyperacute T waves, T wave inversion, or transient intraventricular conduction defects such as bundle branch or fascicular block may be evident.

3. While it can occur in normal arteries (it may be seen at coronary angiography on cannulating the right coronary artery, and cocaine is a potent stimulus), in 90 per cent of patients coronary artery vasospasm occurs at the site of atheroma. ST segment elevation may suggest an acute myocardial infarction, but with resolution of chest pain, the ST segments return to normal. It usually occurs at rest. Patients may also report symptoms of Raynaud's phenomenon. The patient in this case had been using cannabis prior to admission.

4. Treatment for Prinzmetal's (vasospastic) angina should include a calcium channel blocker and/or a nitrate.

COMMENTARY

- Prinzmetal's or variant angina occurs almost exclusively at rest, is not usually brought on by exertion or emotion, and is associated with ST segment elevation which can occur in any lead – the risk of sudden death is increased if seen in both anterior and inferior leads. It may be associated with myocardial infarction and cardiac arrhythmias, including ventricular tachycardia, ventricular fibrillation and sudden death.

- Variant angina tends to affect younger patients than does chronic stable angina or unstable angina. Most will have few conventional risk factors other than smoking. Illicit drug use with cannabis, a potent coronary vasoconstrictor and platelet activator, and cocaine, which causes alpha adrenergically mediated coronary constriction when 'snorted', should always be considered in a young person with severe chest pain, ST segment elevation and few risk factors.

- In patients prone to coronary artery spasm, coronary artery tone and responsiveness to constrictor stimuli are increased. A number of provocative tests have been developed, the most sensitive being ergonovine, an ergot alkaloid that stimulates alpha adrenergic and serotonin receptors which have a direct vasoconstrictive effect on vascular smooth muscle. It may be administered when coronary angiography has demonstrated normal coronary arteries. Hyperventilation is only slightly less sensitive than ergonovine. Most patients have underlying coronary disease and spasm tends to occur close to existing coronary lesions.

- Treatment is based on relieving the coronary spasm:
  - calcium channel blockers
  - nitrates

- Beta blockers may *worsen* coronary spasm and should be avoided.

Further reading

Making Sense of the ECG 4th edition: Prinzmetal's (vasospastic) angina, p 166.

CASE 51

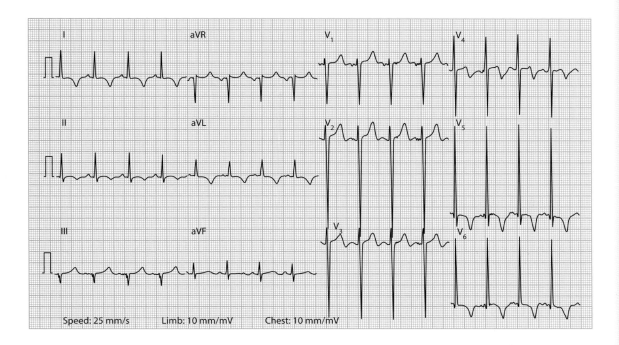

Speed: 25 mm/s   Limb: 10 mm/mV   Chest: 10 mm/mV

CLINICAL SCENARIO

Male, aged 55 years.

Presenting complaint
Syncopal episode while walking uphill.

History of presenting complaint
Three-month history of gradually worsening breathlessness and dizziness on exertion, culminating in a brief syncopal episode while walking uphill. An ambulance was called and the patient was brought to the hospital where this ECG was recorded.

Past medical history
Nil.

Examination
Patient comfortable at rest. Alert and oriented.
Pulse: 96/min, regular, slow rising.
Blood pressure: 108/86.
JVP: not elevated.
Precordium: left parasternal heave.
Heart sounds: loud (4/6) ejection systolic murmur heard in the aortic area, radiating to both carotid arteries.
Chest auscultation: unremarkable.
No peripheral oedema.

Investigations
FBC: Hb 13.8, WCC 7.1, platelets 388.
U&E: Na 141, K 4.4, urea 6.8, creatinine 112.
Chest X-ray: normal heart size, clear lung fields.

QUESTIONS

1. What does this ECG show?
2. What investigation would help to confirm this?
3. What can cause these appearances? What is the likely cause here?
4. What are the treatment options?

ECG ANALYSIS

Rate	96/min
Rhythm	Sinus rhythm
QRS axis	Normal (+11°)
P waves	Normal
PR interval	Normal (160 ms)
QRS duration	Normal (80 ms)
T waves	Inverted in leads I, aVL, V4–V6, and also in lead II
QTc interval	Prolonged (500 ms)

Additional comments

There are very deep S waves (up to 48 mm) in leads V2–V3 and very tall R waves (up to 44 mm) in leads V5–V6.

ANSWERS

1. This ECG shows very deep S waves (up to 48 mm) in leads V2–V3 and very tall R waves (up to 44 mm) in leads V5–V6, together with inverted T waves in leads I, aVL, V4–V6 (and also in lead II). These appearances are indicative of left ventricular hypertrophy with 'strain'.

2. An echocardiogram (or cardiac magnetic resonance scan) would allow direct visualization of the left ventricle, assessment of the extent of left ventricular hypertrophy, assessment of left ventricular systolic (and diastolic) function, and also assessment of the structure and function of the aortic valve.

3. Left ventricular hypertrophy can result from:
   - hypertension
   - aortic stenosis
   - coarctation of the aorta
   - hypertrophic cardiomyopathy.

   The clinical findings indicate that aortic stenosis is the most likely cause of left ventricular hypertrophy in this case.

4. Where left ventricular hypertrophy is secondary to pressure overload of the left ventricle, the appropriate treatment is that of the underlying cause. In the case of aortic stenosis, the aortic valve must be assessed by echocardiography (or cardiac magnetic resonance scanning) and, if severe symptomatic aortic stenosis is confirmed, make plans for aortic valve replacement.

COMMENTARY

- The diagnostic ECG criteria for left ventricular hypertrophy were discussed earlier in Case 35. The ECG in the present case meets several of these diagnostic criteria:
  - R wave of 25 mm or more in the left chest leads
  - S wave of 25 mm or more in the right chest leads
  - Sum of S wave in lead V1 and R wave in lead V5 or V6 greater than 35 mm (Sokolow–Lyon criteria)
  - Sum of tallest R wave and deepest S wave in the chest leads greater than 45 mm.
  - The Cornell criteria are met:
    - The Cornell criteria involve measuring the S wave in lead V3 and the R wave in lead aVL. Left ventricular hypertrophy is indicated by a sum of >28 mm in men and >20 mm in women.
  - The ECG also meets the Romhilt–Estes criteria for left ventricular hypertrophy, scoring 6 points:
    - S wave in right chest leads of 25 mm or more, and also R wave in left chest leads of 25 mm or more (3 points)
    - ST segment and T wave changes ('typical strain') in a patient not taking digitalis (3 points).
- The presence of ST segment depression and/or T wave inversion in the context of left ventricular hypertrophy are taken to indicate left ventricular 'strain'. However, it is important to assess the clinical context – ST/T wave changes, particularly if dynamic, associated with symptoms of chest pain may instead indicate myocardial ischaemia.
- The risk of myocardial infarction and stroke in patients with left ventricular hypertrophy with a strain pattern is approximately double that of patients who have left ventricular hypertrophy without strain.

Further reading

Making Sense of the ECG 4th edition: Left ventricular hypertrophy, p 146; Ventricular hypertrophy with 'strain', p 176.

Bauml MA, Underwood DA. Left ventricular hypertrophy: An overlooked cardiovascular risk factor. *Cleveland Clinic J Med* 2010; **77**: 381–7.

CASE 52

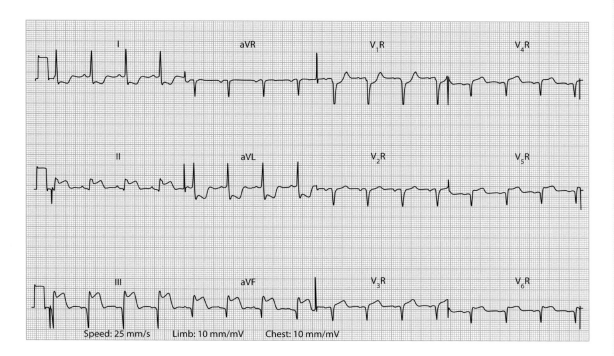

Speed: 25 mm/s   Limb: 10 mm/mV   Chest: 10 mm/mV

CLINICAL SCENARIO

Male, aged 64 years.

Presenting complaint
Severe chest pain ('tight band' around chest), associated with breathlessness. Felt dizzy and fainted.

History of presenting complaint
Digging in garden all day. Ignored chest pain earlier in day.

Past medical history
High blood pressure for several years.
Was a heavy smoker until 4 weeks ago.
Strong family history of coronary artery disease.

Examination
Pulse: 90/min, regular.
Blood pressure: 92/70.
JVP: elevated by 3 cm.
Heart sounds: normal.
Chest auscultation: unremarkable.
Mild peripheral oedema.

Investigations
FBC: Hb 14.4, WCC 11.2, platelets 332.
U&E: Na 143, K 4.6, urea 5.4, creatinine 108.
Troponin I: elevated at 2355 (after 6 h).
Chest X-ray: normal heart size, clear lung fields.
Echocardiogram: normal valve function. Inferior hypokinesia of left ventricle (ejection fraction 48 per cent); right ventricle – impaired function.

QUESTIONS

1. What sort of ECG recording is this?
2. What does this ECG show?
3. What treatment would be appropriate in this patient?

ECG ANALYSIS

Rate	90/min
Rhythm	Sinus rhythm
QRS axis	Normal (+20°)
P waves	Normal
PR interval	Normal (160 ms)
QRS duration	Normal (110 ms)
T waves	Normal
QTc interval	Prolonged (490 ms)

Additional comments

There is inferior ST segment elevation with reciprocal lateral ST segment depression. The right-sided chest leads show ST segment elevation in leads V3R–V6R.

ANSWERS

1. This is an ECG showing the usual limb leads but **right-sided chest leads** (V1R–V6R). Perform an ECG with right-sided chest leads in all patients presenting with an acute inferior myocardial infarction, to look for evidence of right ventricular involvement (as shown by ST segment elevation in lead V4R).

2. The ECG shows an **acute inferior STEMI** (ST segment elevation in leads II, III, aVF) with reciprocal ST segment depression laterally (leads I and aVL). There is ST segment elevation in leads V3R–V6R. The presence of ST segment elevation in lead V4R is indicative of **right ventricular involvement**.

3. Aspirin 300 mg orally (then 75 mg once daily), clopidogrel 300 mg orally (then 75 mg once daily), glyceryl trinitrate sublingually, pain relief (intravenous opiate, plus an anti-emetic), oxygen if hypoxic. Prompt restoration of myocardial blood flow is required with primary percutaneous coronary intervention (PCI) or, if primary PCI is not available, thrombolysis. In right ventricular infarction, hypotension may be the result of reduced left ventricular filling pressures (as a result of right ventricular impairment) and so careful fluid management is essential.

COMMENTARY

- The prognosis in inferior myocardial infarction is generally very good. However, when the infarction involves the right ventricle (about 50 per cent of cases), the risk of severe complications is increased almost sixfold:
  - death, ventricular fibrillation, re-infarction.
  - risk of right-sided heart failure (elevated JVP, peripheral oedema, low output state but with no evidence of pulmonary oedema).

- In inferior myocardial infarction with right ventricular involvement, hypotension is usually due to poor right ventricular contractility secondary to the right ventricular infarction. Volume expansion with aliquots of 250 mL of normal saline intravenously, repeated as necessary, may be effective in maintaining right ventricular output and thus left ventricular filling pressure. Failure to respond warrants consideration of right- and left-sided filling pressure monitoring using a Swan–Ganz catheter – high right-sided pressures and a low pulmonary capillary wedge (= left atrial) pressure confirms right ventricular infarction. It is essential to avoid vasodilator drugs which may reduce the right ventricular output even further.

Further reading

Making Sense of the ECG 4th edition: ST segment elevation myocardial infarction, p 160; Why is right ventricular infarction important? p 165.

Chockalingam A, Gnanavelu G, Subramaniam, T. Right ventricular myocardial infarction: presentation and acute outcomes. *Angiology* 2005; **56**: 371–6.

CASE 53

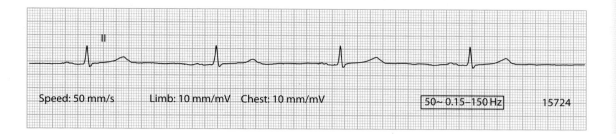

Speed: 50 mm/s   Limb: 10 mm/mV   Chest: 10 mm/mV   50~ 0.15–150 Hz   15724

CLINICAL SCENARIO

Male, aged 22 years.

Presenting complaint
Fatigue.

History of presenting complaint
Longstanding history of fatigue.
No other associated symptoms.

Past medical history
Childhood asthma – no longer uses inhalers.

Examination
Pulse: 58/min, regular.
Blood pressure: 124/76.
JVP: not elevated.
Heart sounds: normal.
Chest auscultation: unremarkable.
No peripheral oedema.

Investigations
FBC: Hb 15.5, WCC 5.2, platelets 389.
U&E: Na 143, K 4.9, urea 3.6, creatinine 67.
Thyroid function: normal.

QUESTIONS

1. What does this ECG show?
2. What would you do next?
3. What is the cause of this patient's fatigue?

ECG ANALYSIS

Rate	58/min
Rhythm	Sinus rhythm (slight bradycardia)
QRS axis	Unable to assess (single lead)
P waves	Present
PR interval	Normal (160 ms)
QRS duration	Normal (80 ms)
T waves	Normal
QTc interval	Normal (413 ms)

Additional comments

The paper speed is set at 50 mm/s, double the normal recording speed.

ANSWERS

1. This ECG shows normal sinus rhythm with a heart rate of 58/min (slight bradycardia). At first glance, the rate looks like it might be slower than that (29/min), but that is because the recording has been made at double the normal paper speed (50 mm/s rather than the standard 25 mm/s). The paper speed is shown at the lower left corner of the rhythm strip.
2. Repeat the ECG at the standard paper setting of 25 mm/s.
3. This ECG rhythm strip does not reveal an explanation for this patient's fatigue – his heart rate is virtually normal at 58/min. Further clinical assessment is required to identify the cause of his fatigue.

COMMENTARY

- The standard ECG paper speed in the UK and the US is 25 mm/s, which makes each small square equivalent to 0.04 s and each large square equivalent to 0.2 s. By counting large and/or small squares, you can calculate such parameters as heart rate and PR and QT intervals.
- If a 'non-standard' paper speed is used, the 'time value' of small and large squares need to be adjusted accordingly. At 50 mm/s, the small squares will equal 0.02 s and the large squares 0.1 s. All measurements and calculations must take the new speed setting into account.
- A speed setting of 50 mm/s is sometimes used to make measurements easier (by doubling the width of every wave, some features can be seen and/or measured more easily). A paper speed of 50 mm/s is used as the standard setting in some parts of Europe, rather than 25 mm/s.
- Annotate all ECGs with the paper speed that was used for the recording. If a non-standard paper speed was used, highlight this clearly to avoid misinterpretation.
- When an ECG has been recorded using a non-standard paper speed in error, repeat it using the appropriate paper speed.

Further reading

Making Sense of the ECG 4th edition: Performing an ECG recording, p 21; Incorrect paper speed, p 205.
The Society for Cardiological Science and Technology: Clinical Guidelines by Consensus. Recording a standard 12-lead electrocardiogram: an approved methodology. February 2010. Available for download from www.scst.org.uk

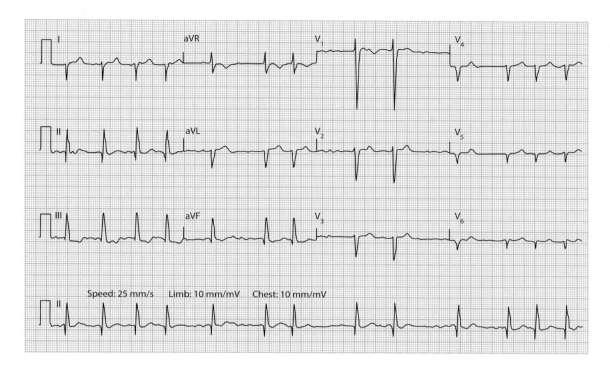

Speed: 25 mm/s   Limb: 10 mm/mV   Chest: 10 mm/mV

CLINICAL SCENARIO

Male, aged 22 years.

Presenting complaint
Admitted with lower respiratory tract infection.

History of presenting complaint
Cough, productive of blood-stained sputum; fever; tachycardia

Past medical history
Nil of note.

Examination
Pulse: 76/min, irregularly irregular.
Blood pressure: 134/76.

JVP: not elevated.
Heart sounds: quiet; heard best on right side of chest.
Chest auscultation: bronchial breathing right lower lobe.
No peripheral oedema.

Investigations
FBC: Hb 15.6, WCC 13.5, platelets 224.
U&E: Na 139, K 3.9, urea 4.4, creatinine 86.
Chest X-ray: dextrocardia; consolidation right lower lobe.
Echocardiogram: dextrocardia. Normal valves. Left ventricular function normal (ejection fraction 67 per cent).

QUESTIONS

1. What abnormalities does this ECG show?
2. What are the likely causes?
3. What are the key issues in managing this patient?

ECG ANALYSIS

Rate	76/min
Rhythm	Atrial fibrillation
QRS axis	Extreme right axis deviation (+124°)
P waves	Absent (atrial fibrillation)
PR interval	N/A
QRS duration	Normal (112 ms)
T waves	Normal
QTc interval	Normal (446 ms)

Additional comments

There is a decrease in QRS complex size from lead V1 to lead V6.

ANSWERS

1. The rhythm is atrial fibrillation. Leads I and aVL are negative and leads II, III and aVR are positive – this is extreme right axis deviation. The R waves are generally small across the chest leads, and decrease in size from V1 to V6 (normally, the R waves are small in V1, equipolar at V3 or V4 and largest at V6).

2. This is **dextrocardia**. Dextrocardia is a naturally occurring anomaly, seen in 1:10 000 people. The ECG 'abnormalities' occur because the recording reflects the heart's abnormal position in the thorax. The ECG will 'normalize' if the chest leads are reversed so that lead V1 is recorded from the *left* sternal edge and V6 from the *right* axilla. The patient's atrial fibrillation is likely to have been triggered by the lower respiratory tract infection, but always undertake a careful review for other possible causes.

3. The ECG 'abnormalities' seen in dextrocardia must not be considered pathological – the heart is usually structurally normal. It is important that the finding of dextrocardia be recorded prominently in a patient's notes to prevent mishaps. Manage the patient's atrial fibrillation in the same way as any other patient with atrial fibrillation (see Case 6).

COMMENTARY

- The term *situs* describes the position of the cardiac atria and viscera, cardiac situs being determined by atrial location, so:
  - situs solitus – is the normal orientation of viscera and a left-sided heart
  - situs inversus – is reversal of all the major structures in the thorax and abdomen
  - situs ambiguous – the orientation of heart and viscera conform to neither situs solitus nor inversus (any structure with a right-left asymmetry can be normal, completely reversed or neither).
- In situs inversus with levocardia, the apex of the heart points to the left; with dextrocardia, it points to the right. Dextrocardia on its own is known as situs solitus with dextrocardia.
- Other congenital cardiovascular abnormalities can be associated with dextrocardia, such as single ventricle, atrial or ventricular septal defects, anomalous pulmonary venous return, and transposition of the great arteries. When dextrocardia occurs with just the heart incorrectly positioned, functionally significant complex cardiac abnormalities are more likely.
- Situs inversus totalis may be associated with ciliary dysfunction (Kartagener's syndrome) in which patients experience repeated sinus and respiratory infections resulting in bronchiectasis, chronic sinusitis and nasal polyposis. Life expectancy is normal if bronchiectasis is adequately treated.

Further reading

Making Sense of the ECG 4th edition: Dextrocardia, p 149.

CASE 55

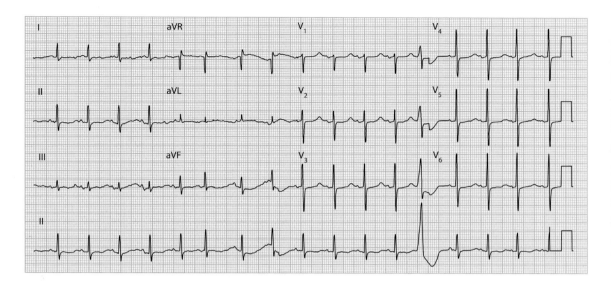

CLINICAL SCENARIO

Female, aged 73 years.

Presenting complaint
Asymptomatic.

History of presenting complaint
Asymptomatic. Routine ECG performed as a pre-operative assessment.

Past medical history
Osteoarthritis (awaiting knee surgery).

Examination
Pulse: 102/min, irregular (ectopic beats).
Blood pressure: 138/84.
JVP: not elevated.
Heart sounds: normal.
Chest auscultation: unremarkable.
No peripheral oedema.

Investigations
FBC: Hb 13.9, WCC 7.8, platelets 255.
U&E: Na 139, K 4.4, urea 7.4, creatinine 102.
Chest X-ray: normal heart size, clear lung fields.
Echocardiogram: normal.

QUESTIONS

1. What does this ECG show?
2. What can cause this abnormality?

ECG ANALYSIS

Rate	102/min
Rhythm	Sinus rhythm with an atrial and a ventricular ectopic beat
QRS axis	Normal (+27°)
P waves	Normal
PR interval	Normal (160 ms)
QRS duration	Normal (80 ms)
T waves	Normal
QTc interval	Prolonged (574 ms)

ANSWERS

1. This ECG shows a very prolonged QTc interval of 574 ms.
2. Causes of QTc prolongation include:
   - long QT syndrome
   - drug effects
   - hypocalcaemia
   - acute myocarditis.

   QTc prolongation can sometimes also be seen in cases of acute myocardial infarction, cerebral injury, hypertrophic cardiomyopathy and hypothermia.

COMMENTARY

- The normal QT interval varies with heart rate, becoming shorter at faster rates. Measurements of the QT interval therefore need to be corrected for heart rate. The most common method for calculating the corrected QT interval (QTc) is Bazett's formula, dividing the measured QT interval by the square root of the RR interval (all measurements in seconds).
- Bazett's formula has limitations, however, and tends to overcorrect or undercorrect the QT interval at extremes of heart rate. Other formulae are also used, and so-called linear formulae tend to be more uniform over a wide range of heart rates.
- QT intervals tend to be a little longer in women than in men, and so a normal QTc is up to 450 ms in men and 460 ms in women. Long QT intervals are associated with a risk of polymorphic ventricular tachycardia (torsades de pointes), which is discussed in Case 61.
- Many hereditary syndromes are now recognized in which an abnormality of the sodium or potassium ion channels causes a susceptibility to ventricular arrhythmias and sudden cardiac death. These syndromes include long QT syndrome (LQTS), in which genetic abnormalities of the potassium or sodium channels lead to prolonged ventricular repolarization and hence prolongation of the QT interval.
- Several genetic abnormalities have now been identified, the three most common being termed LQT1 and LQT2 (potassium channel abnormalities) and LQT3 (sodium channel abnormality).
- Several anti-arrhythmic drugs cause prolongation of the QT interval by slowing myocardial conduction, and thus repolarization. Examples are quinidine, procainamide and flecainide. QT interval prolongation is also seen with terfenadine and tricyclic antidepressants.

Further reading

Making Sense of the ECG 4th edition: Is the QTc interval long? p 192.

Goldenberg I, Moss AJ. Long QT syndrome. *J Am Coll Cardiol* 2008; **51**: 2291–300.

Rautaharju PM, Surawicz B, Gettes LS. AHA/ACCF/HRS recommendations for the standardization and interpretation of the electrocardiogram: Part IV: The ST segment, T and U waves, and the QT interval. *J Am Coll Cardiol* 2009; **53**: 982–91.

CASE 56

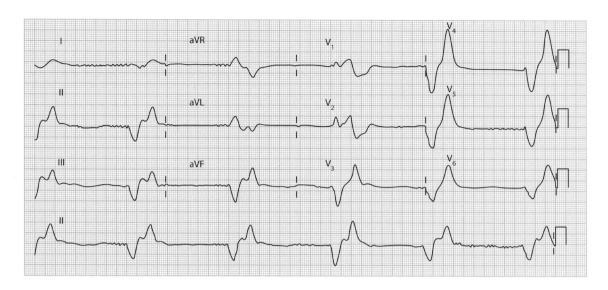

CLINICAL SCENARIO

Male, aged 72 years.

Presenting complaint
Severe central chest pain.

History of presenting complaint
Patient currently an inpatient on the coronary care unit. He had an acute myocardial infarction 36 h previously.

Past medical history
Hypertension.
Type 2 diabetes mellitus.

Examination
Pulse: 36/min, regular.
Blood pressure: 124/88.
JVP: not elevated.
Heart sounds: normal.
Chest auscultation: unremarkable.
No peripheral oedema.

Investigations
FBC: Hb 12.4, WCC 9.6, platelets 256.
U&E: Na 139, K 4.1, urea 4.3, creatinine 128.
Troponin I: elevated at 5425 (after 6 h).
Chest X-ray: mild cardiomegaly, early pulmonary congestion.
Echocardiogram: left ventricular function mildly impaired (ejection fraction 47 per cent).

QUESTIONS

1. What does this ECG show?
2. What is the mechanism of this?
3. What are the likely causes?
4. What are the key issues in managing this patient?

ECG ANALYSIS

Rate	36/min
Rhythm	Regular
QRS axis	Left axis deviation (–90°)
P waves	Absent
PR interval	N/A
QRS duration	Prolonged (220 ms)
T waves	Normal
QTc interval	Prolonged (464 ms)

ANSWERS

1. The QRS complexes are wide and appear in a regular rhythm. This is a 'slow' form of monomorphic ventricular 'tachycardia', sometimes called 'idioventricular rhythm' or 'accelerated idioventricular rhythm'.
2. Idioventricular rhythm is caused by enhanced automaticity of His–Purkinje fibres or myocardium, appearing under specific metabolic conditions such as acute myocardial ischaemia (the most common). Other causes include electrolyte abnormalities (which may require correction), myocarditis, cardiomyopathy and following cardiac arrest.
3. It is usually seen in the first two days after an acute myocardial infarction. When seen after thrombolysis, it is usually accepted as a marker of successful coronary reperfusion.
4. The rhythm abnormality is benign and treatment is necessary only if there is haemodynamic compromise.

COMMENTARY

- Sometimes called 'slow VT', idioventricular rhythm:
  - is a benign form of ventricular tachycardia
  - it is equally common in inferior and anterior myocardial infarction
  - often occurs as an escape rhythm during slowing of the sinus rate
  - usually has a rate of 60–120/min with a QRS complex duration >120 ms (in the case presented here, the rate is significantly lower).
- Rarely, the ventricular rate may increase, causing ventricular tachycardia or ventricular fibrillation. Treatment then involves increasing the sinus rate with atropine or atrial pacing.

Further reading

Making Sense of the ECG 4th edition: Accelerated idioventricular rhythm, p 82.

CASE 57

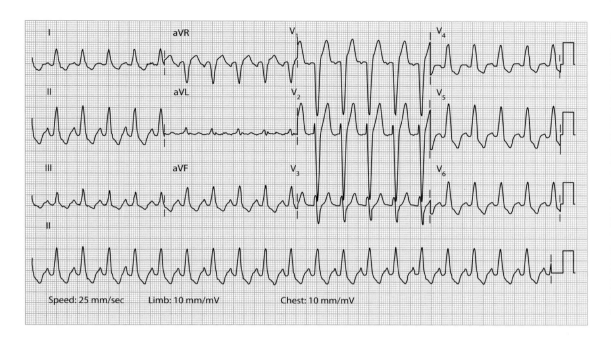

Speed: 25 mm/sec   Limb: 10 mm/mV   Chest: 10 mm/mV

CLINICAL SCENARIO

Female, aged 77 years.

Presenting complaint
Haematemesis and melaena.

History of presenting complaint
Patient had been taking non-steroidal anti-inflammatory drugs for the past 4 weeks to obtain pain relief from her osteoarthritis. She presented with haematemesis, having vomited approximately 500 mL of fresh blood, and subsequently developed melaena.

Past medical history
Osteoarthritis.
Ischaemic heart disease.

Examination
Clammy, pale.
Pulse: 120/min, regular.
Blood pressure: 86/46.
JVP: not seen.
Heart sounds: normal.
Chest auscultation: unremarkable.
No peripheral oedema.

Investigations
FBC: Hb 6.8, WCC 13.2, platelets 309.
U&E: Na 137, K 4.1, urea 16.7, creatinine 93.
Chest X-ray: normal heart size, clear lung fields.
Gastroscopy: large, actively bleeding duodenal ulcer.

QUESTIONS

1. What does this ECG show?
2. What would you do about the heart rate?

ECG ANALYSIS

Rate	120/min
Rhythm	Sinus tachycardia
QRS axis	Normal (+48°)
P waves	Present
PR interval	Normal (120 ms)
QRS duration	Broad (130 ms)
T waves	Normal
QTc interval	Normal (450 ms)

Additional comments

The QRS complexes have a left bundle branch block morphology.

ANSWERS

1. This ECG shows a tachycardia (heart rate 120/min) with broad QRS complexes (QRS duration 130 ms). The QRS complexes have a left bundle branch block (LBBB) morphology. On careful inspection, P waves can be seen before the QRS complexes – the P waves are most easily seen in lead V1. This broad-complex tachycardia is therefore sinus tachycardia with aberrant conduction (LBBB).

2. This patient's sinus tachycardia is appropriate to her haemodynamic state – she has lost blood and is hypotensive, and has therefore developed a sinus tachycardia to help maintain cardiac output. Trying to slow down the tachycardia in these circumstances would be dangerous, causing haemodynamic decompensation. The management of sinus tachycardia therefore depends critically on the identification and, where possible, treatment of the underlying cause. The appropriate action here would be to correct the hypovolaemia and to prevent any further blood loss.

COMMENTARY

- Broad-complex tachycardia (QRS complex duration >120 ms) can result from:
  - ventricular tachycardia (VT)
  - supraventricular tachycardia (SVT) with aberrant conduction
  - ventricular pacing.
- If a patient has a pre-existing bundle branch block in normal sinus rhythm, that bundle branch block will also remain present during episodes of SVT. However, some patients may have normal QRS complexes while in normal sinus rhythm, but develop a bundle branch block only during episodes of tachycardia ('functional' bundle branch block). In such cases, the development of functional right bundle branch block (RBBB) is more common than functional LBBB. Sudden changes in RR interval (as seen, for example, in atrial fibrillation) are particularly likely to cause functional bundle branch block – this is referred to as the Ashman phenomenon.
- SVT with aberrant conduction also includes SVT occurring with ventricular preexcitation, for example antidromic atrioventricular re-entry tachycardia or atrial fibrillation with pre-excitation, both of which can occur in Wolff–Parkinson–White syndrome (see Case 59).
- Distinguishing between VT and SVT with aberrant conduction can be challenging. If the QRS morphology has a typical RBBB or LBBB, then it is likely to be SVT with aberrant conduction. However, this is certainly not diagnostic as some forms of VT can resemble LBBB or RBBB very closely. If the QRS complexes are very broad (RBBB morphology with QRS duration >140 ms, LBBB morphology with QRS duration >160 ms), then VT is more likely. An extreme QRS axis (between –90° and –180°) also points towards VT, as do concordant negative QRS complexes in the chest leads. One of the most valuable criteria for diagnosing VT is the presence of independent atrial activity (see Commentary, Case 58).
- Broad-complex tachycardia should always be managed as VT until proven otherwise.

Further reading

Making Sense of the ECG 4th edition: Sinus tachycardia, p 55; How do I distinguish between VT and SVT? p 86; Bundle branch block, p 153.

Eckardt L, Breithardt G, Kirchhof, P. Approach to wide complex tachycardias in patients without structural heart disease. Heart 2006; **92**: 704–11.

CASE 58

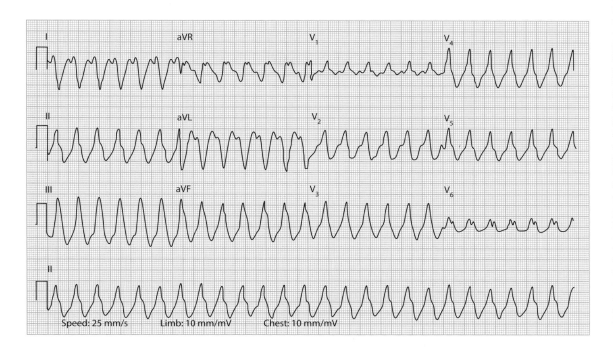

Speed: 25 mm/s   Limb: 10 mm/mV   Chest: 10 mm/mV

CLINICAL SCENARIO

Male, aged 76 years.

Presenting complaint
Chest pain and breathlessness.

History of presenting complaint
Patient was woken from sleep by severe chest pain and breathlessness.

Past medical history
Myocardial infarction 12 months previously. Treated with thrombolysis. Occasional chest pain on exertion at intervals since. Had reduced activities to avoid chest pain.

Examination
Pulse: 152/min, regular.

Blood pressure: 108/72.
JVP: not elevated.
Heart sounds: normal.
Chest auscultation: unremarkable.
No peripheral oedema.

Investigations
FBC: Hb 12.8, WCC 6.3, platelets 267.
U&E: Na 135, K 3.2, urea 8.2, creatinine 138.
Thyroid function: normal.
Troponin I: negative.
Chest X-ray: marked cardiomegaly with signs of pulmonary congestion.
Echocardiogram: moderate mitral regurgitation into moderately dilated left atrium. Left ventricular function severely impaired (ejection fraction 25 per cent).

QUESTIONS

1. What does this ECG show?
2. What are the key issues in managing this patient?

ECG ANALYSIS

Rate	152/min
Rhythm	Ventricular tachycardia
QRS axis	+93°
P waves	Not seen
PR interval	N/A
QRS duration	Prolonged (164 ms)
T waves	Not clearly seen
QTc interval	T waves not clearly seen

ANSWERS

1. This ECG shows a broad-complex tachycardia. There is positive concordance of the anterior chest leads (the QRS complexes in the anterior leads are all positive). This is **monomorphic ventricular tachycardia** (VT).

2. Acute management:
   - Cardiopulmonary resuscitation – if the patient is haemodynamically compromised, follow the appropriate life support protocols including electrical cardioversion as appropriate.
   - Manage the underlying cause (e.g. acute coronary syndrome) as appropriate.

3. Long-term management:
   - Following the initial management and correction of VT, longer-term management should be discussed with a cardiologist.
   - Long-term prophylaxis is usually not necessary for VT occurring within the first 48 h following an acute myocardial infarction.
   - Where prophylaxis is needed, effective drug treatments include sotalol (particularly when VT is exercise related) or amiodarone.
   - VT related to bradycardia should be treated by pacing.
   - Ablation or surgery can be used to remove a ventricular focus or re-entry circuit identified by electrophysiological testing.
   - Implantable cardioverter defibrillators (ICDs) can be implanted to deliver overdrive pacing and/or shocks for recurrent episodes of VT and VF.

COMMENTARY

- It can be difficult to differentiate VT and SVT with aberrant conduction (if in doubt, always manage as VT until proven otherwise).
- ECG findings favouring VT:
  - a broad complex tachycardia in a patient with a history of coronary disease (especially myocardial infarction)
  - QRS duration in tachycardia – the wider the QRS, the more likely the rhythm is to be VT (VT is the most common cause of tachycardia with a broad QRS)
  - normal QRS duration in sinus rhythm but >140 ms during tachycardia
  - marked change in axis (whether to the left or right), compared with ECG in sinus rhythm
  - concordance – the QRS complexes in the chest leads are all positive or negative.
- Evidence of atrioventricular dissociation is strongly supportive of a diagnosis of VT:
  - independent P wave activity – P waves occurring with no relation to the QRS complexes
  - capture beats – an atrial impulse manages to 'capture' the ventricles for one beat, causing a normal QRS complex, which may be preceded by a P wave
  - fusion beats – these appear when the ventricles are activated by an atrial impulse and a ventricular impulse simultaneously.

Further reading

Making Sense of the ECG 4th edition: Ventricular tachycardia, p 83; How do I distinguish between VT and SVT? p 86.

Alzand BSN, Crijns HJGM. Diagnostic criteria of broad QRS complex tachycardia: decades of evolution. *Europace* 2011; **13**: 465–72.

Brugada P, Brugada J, Mont L *et al*. A new approach to the differential diagnosis of a regular tachycardia with a wide QRS complex. *Circulation* 1991; **83**: 1649–59.

Jastrzebski M, Kukla P, Czarnecka D *et al*. Comparison of five electrocardiographic methods for differentiation of wide QRS-complex tachycardias. *Europace* 2012; **14**: 1165–71.

NICE Guideline TA95 – Implantable cardioverter defibrillators. Available for download from: http://guidance.nice.org.uk/TA95

Vereckei A, Duray G, Szénási G *et al.* Application of a new algorithm in the differential diagnosis of wide QRS complex tachycardia. *Eur Heart J* 2007; **28**: 589–600.

CASE 59

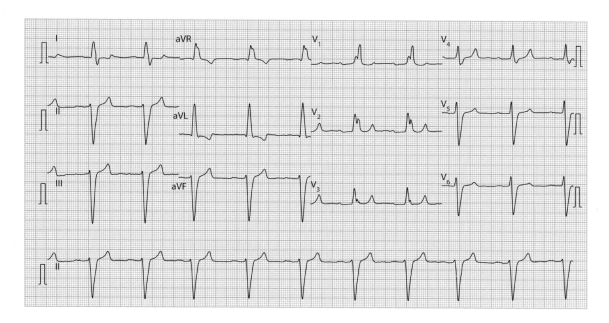

CLINICAL SCENARIO

Female, aged 77 years.

Presenting complaint
Syncope.

History of presenting complaint
Two abrupt syncopal events during the last month.

Past medical history
Angina, hypertension, diabetes mellitus, chronic kidney disease.

Examination
Pulse: 60/min, regular.
Blood pressure: 172/84.
Heart sounds: normal.
Chest auscultation: unremarkable.
No peripheral oedema.

Investigations
FBC: Hb 14.5, WCC 7.2, platelets 353.
U&E: Na 140, K 4.9, urea 10.2, creatinine 156.
Thyroid function: normal.

QUESTIONS

1. What key features are shown on this ECG?
2. What is this condition called?
3. Is this related to the patient's syncope?

ECG ANALYSIS

Rate	60/min
Rhythm	Sinus rhythm
QRS axis	Left axis deviation (−81°)
P waves	Normal
PR interval	Prolonged (266 ms)
QRS duration	Broad complexes (180 ms)
T waves	Biphasic in lead I and inverted in lead aVL
QTc interval	Borderline prolonged (463 ms)

Additional comments

The QRS complexes have a right bundle branch block morphology.

ANSWERS

1. This ECG shows:
   - first-degree atrioventricular block (PR interval 266 ms)
   - left axis deviation (QRS complex axis −81°)
   - right bundle branch block.
2. This combination of conduction abnormalities is called **trifascicular block**.
3. Trifascicular block can progress to third-degree atrioventricular block ('complete heart block'). This can occur intermittently, and may therefore account for the syncopal events.

COMMENTARY

- Many different types of conduction block are possible at different levels of the conduction system, including atrioventricular (AV) block, right bundle branch block (RBBB), left bundle branch block (LBBB), left anterior fascicular block (LAFB) and left posterior fascicular block (LPFB).
- When these blocks occur in combination, the possible permutations include:
  - LAFB + LPFB = LBBB
  - RBBB + LAFB = bifascicular block
  - RBBB + LPFB = bifascicular block
  - RBBB + LAFB + first-degree AV block = trifascicular block
  - RBBB + LPFB + first-degree AV block = trifascicular block
  - RBBB + LBBB = third-degree AV block (complete heart block)
  - RBBB + LAFB + LPFB = third-degree AV block (complete heart block)
- Permanent pacing is indicated when there is bifascicular or trifascicular block with a clear history of syncope, or documented intermittent failure of the remaining fascicle.

Further reading

Making Sense of the ECG 4th edition: Conduction problems, p 93; Pacemakers and implantable cardioverter defibrillators, p 209.

Epstein AE, DiMarco JP, Ellenbogen KA *et al*. ACC/AHA/HRS 2008 guidelines for device-based therapy of cardiac rhythm abnormalities. A Report of the American College of Cardiology/American Heart Association task force on practice guidelines (writing committee to revise the ACC/AHA/NASPE 2002 guideline update for implantation of cardiac pacemakers and antiarrhythmia devices). *J Am Coll Cardiol* 2008; **51**: e1–62.

The Task Force on Cardiac Pacing and Resynchronization Therapy of the European Society of Cardiology (ESC). 2013 ESC guidelines on cardiac pacing and cardiac resynchronization therapy. *Eur Heart J* 2013; **34**: 2281–329.

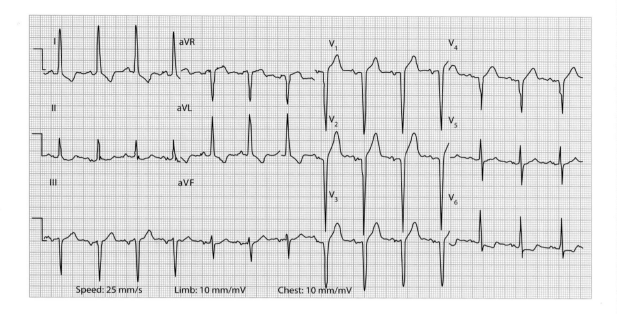

Speed: 25 mm/s   Limb: 10 mm/mV   Chest: 10 mm/mV

CLINICAL SCENARIO

Female, aged 36 years.

Presenting complaint

Breathlessness, intermittent chest pain and palpitations.

History of presenting complaint

Been slowing down a lot recently; had to abandon walking holiday in Scotland as very breathless on attempting to walk up hills.

Past medical history

Non-smoker.
No family history of cardiovascular disease but her sister is undergoing investigations for similar problems.

Examination

Pulse: 84/min, regular.
Blood pressure: 136/86.
JVP: not elevated.
Heart sounds: soft ejection systolic murmur in aortic area and lower left sternal edge.
Chest auscultation: unremarkable.
No peripheral oedema.

Investigations

FBC: Hb 12.9, WCC 7.8, platelets 259
U&E: Na 137, K 4.2, urea 5.3, creatinine 88.
Troponin I: negative.
Chest X-ray: mild cardiomegaly.

QUESTIONS

1. What does this ECG show?
2. What is the mechanism of this?
3. What are the likely causes?
4. What are the key issues in managing this patient?

ECG ANALYSIS

Rate	84/min
Rhythm	Sinus rhythm
QRS axis	Normal (−15°)
P waves	Normal
PR interval	Normal (198 ms)
QRS duration	Normal (100 ms)
T waves	Inverted I, aVL, V6
QTc interval	Normal (450 ms)

Additional comments

There are deep Q waves in the anterior leads.

ANSWERS

1. The deep anterior Q waves are suggestive of septal hypertrophy. Echocardiography confirmed that the patient had severe asymmetrical hypertrophy of the interventricular septum with obstruction to the left ventricular outflow tract – this is **hypertrophic obstructive cardiomyopathy** (HOCM).
2. ECG changes are due to thickened septal muscle – the most common variety of HOCM. If this is in the outflow tract, the Venturi effect of increased blood flow velocity during systole causes systolic anterior motion of mitral valve (and mitral regurgitation).
3. In 70 per cent, there is a genetic mutation in the gene coding for beta myosin, alpha-tropomyosin and troponin T. Inheritance is autosomal dominant, though 50 per cent of cases are sporadic.
4. An accurate diagnosis is important to establish whether there is obstruction to outflow from the left ventricle – the obstructive variety of cardiomyopathy carries a worse prognosis than non-obstructive. Investigate and monitor for rhythm abnormalities and treat with antiarrhythmic drugs as appropriate – high risk patients may benefit from an implantable cardioverter defibrillator (ICD). Beta blockers or verapamil will reduce gradient across the outflow tract and control angina. In patients with more severe symptoms – reduce outflow tract obstruction by septal myomectomy either surgically or by alcohol ablation. Dual chamber pacing may improve symptoms and increase exercise tolerance. Screening of first-degree relatives is important.

COMMENTARY

- Hypertrophic cardiomyopathy is a heterogeneous disease of the sarcomere with at least 150 different mutations in 10 different sarcomeric proteins. Certain mutations may delay penetrance so that the disease presents late (>60 years). Molecular genetic studies will become more widely available in future to assist diagnosis.
- The 12-lead ECG is abnormal in at least 75 per cent of cases of hypertrophic cardiomyopathy. It may show a mild degree of hypertrophy, or show left ventricular hypertrophy and 'strain', or sharply negative T waves in precordial leads V1–V3, deep Q waves, atrial fibrillation, ventricular ectopics or ventricular tachycardia. ECG changes are often evident before echocardiographic features, especially in the young.
- Characteristic features to look for on echocardiography – asymmetrical left ventricular hypertrophy, small left ventricular cavity, systolic anterior motion of the mitral valve, mitral regurgitation, and mid-systolic closure of the aortic valve.
- Magnetic resonance imaging may be helpful in establishing the diagnosis.
- On identifying the index case, arrange a 12-lead ECG and echocardiogram for first-degree relatives.
- Factors associated with a poor prognosis:
  - personal history of sudden cardiac death events, ventricular fibrillation or sustained ventricular tachycardia
  - personal history of sudden cardiac death events
  - unexplained syncope
  - documented non-sustained ventricular tachycardia
  - maximal left ventricular wall thickness ≥3 cm.

Further reading

Making Sense of the ECG 4th edition: Left ventricular hypertrophy, p 146.

Gersh BJ, Maron BJ, Bonow RO *et al.* 2011 ACCF/AHA guideline for the diagnosis and treatment of hypertrophic cardiomyopathy: a report of the American College of Cardiology Foundation/American Heart Association Task Force on Practice Guidelines. *J Am Coll Cardiol* 2011; **58:** e212– 60.

CASE 61

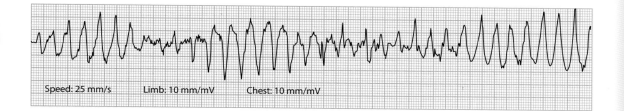

Speed: 25 mm/s   Limb: 10 mm/mV   Chest: 10 mm/mV

CLINICAL SCENARIO

Female, aged 63 years.

Presenting complaint
Syncope.

History of presenting complaint
Patient admitted to hospital complaining of fatigue and muscle weakness after a week's history of diarrhoea and vomiting. She had a syncopal event shortly after admission and ECG monitoring was commenced. Shortly afterwards the patient had another syncopal episode and this ECG was recorded.

Past medical history
Alcoholic cirrhosis of the liver.

Examination
Clinical features of alcoholic liver disease with ascites.
Pulse: too fast to record manually.
Blood pressure: 96/54.
JVP: elevated by 6 cm.
Heart sounds: gallop rhythm.
Chest auscultation: bilateral pleural effusions.
Moderate peripheral oedema.

Investigations
FBC: Hb 10.8, WCC 18.1, platelets 124.
U&E: Na 127, K 2.3, urea 4.9, creatinine 85.
Magnesium: 0.61 mmol/L (normal range 0.7–1.0 mmol/L).
Chest X-ray: small bilateral pleural effusions.

QUESTIONS

1. What rhythm is shown on this rhythm strip?
2. What is the likely cause of this arrhythmia?
3. What treatment would be appropriate?

ECG ANALYSIS

Rate	230/min
Rhythm	Polymorphic ventricular tachycardia
QRS axis	Varying
P waves	Not visible
PR interval	–
QRS duration	Broad
T waves	Not visible
QTc interval	Not measurable on this rhythm strip (but was prolonged at 510 ms on admission 12-lead ECG)

ANSWERS

1. **Polymorphic ventricular tachycardia** (VT), which in the setting of a prolonged QT interval is commonly referred to as **torsades de pointes**.
2. The prolonged QT interval predisposes to polymorphic VT. In this patient's case the likely aetiology of the QT interval prolongation is the electrolyte abnormalities (hypokalaemia and hypomagnesaemia).
3. The electrolyte abnormalities need to be corrected. Follow standard adult life support protocols.

COMMENTARY

- Polymorphic VT is distinguished by a varying QRS complex morphology.
- Polymorphic VT falls into two distinct categories based upon the duration of the QT interval (measured during sinus rhythm):
  - polymorphic VT in the setting of a normal QT interval
  - polymorphic VT in the setting of a prolonged QT interval
- When the underlying QT interval is normal, polymorphic VT may be due to myocardial ischaemia/infarction, coronary reperfusion (following myocardial infarction), structural heart disease or the rare condition of catecholaminergic polymorphic VT.
- When polymorphic VT is seen in the context of a prolonged QT interval, it is commonly called torsades de pointes ('twisting of the points'). There are several causes of QT interval prolongation, including hypocalcaemia, acute myocarditis, long QT syndrome and certain drugs.
- Polymorphic VT carries a risk of precipitating ventricular fibrillation and so urgent assessment (with involvement of a cardiologist) is warranted. In an emergency, follow standard adult life support protocols including urgent defibrillation if required. Treat underlying causes, such as myocardial ischaemia/infarction or electrolyte abnormalities, and stop any causative drugs.
- If the underlying QT interval is prolonged, useful measures can also include the administration of intravenous magnesium and consideration of temporary transvenous pacing (which increases the heart rate and thereby shortens the QT interval). In the longer term, an implantable cardioverter defibrillator may be required if the patient is judged to be at high risk of recurrent arrhythmias and sudden cardiac death.

Further reading

Making Sense of the ECG 4th edition: Polymorphic ventricular tachycardia, p 89; Is the QTc interval long? p 192.

Yap YG, Camm AJ. Drug induced QT prolongation and torsades de pointes. *Heart* 2003; **89**: 1363–72.

CASE 62

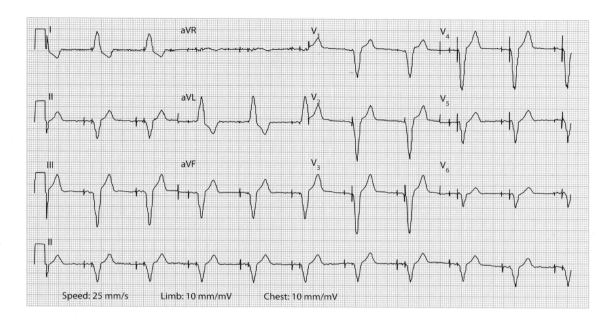

Speed: 25 mm/s   Limb: 10 mm/mV   Chest: 10 mm/mV

CLINICAL SCENARIO

Female, aged 71 years.

Presenting complaint
No specific complaints.

History of presenting complaint
Patient had been diagnosed with complete heart block a few years ago when she presented with dizziness and fatigue. Attended family doctor surgery for routine 'well woman' check and was concerned when ECG performed by the practice nurse was shown to a doctor.

Past medical history
Angina, hypertension, diabetes mellitus. Had experienced feeling weak and dizzy last year – fractured her hip following a fall but now fully independent again.

Examination
Pulse: 60/min, regular.
Blood pressure: 146/90.
JVP: not elevated.
Heart sounds: normal.
Chest auscultation: unremarkable.
Peripheral oedema: nil.

Investigations
FBC: Hb 10.5, WCC 3.9, platelets 145.
U&E: Na 133, K 4.8, urea 5.9, creatinine 129.
Chest X-ray: normal heart size, clear lung fields.
Echocardiogram: mild mitral regurgitation into mildly dilated left atrium. Left ventricular function mildly impaired (ejection fraction 51 per cent).

QUESTIONS

1. What does this ECG show?
2. What is the mechanism of this?
3. What are the likely causes?
4. What are the key issues in managing this patient?

ECG ANALYSIS

Rate	60/min
Rhythm	Atrial and ventricular sequential pacing
QRS axis	Left axis deviation (−61°)
P waves	Very small, visible just after the atrial pacing 'spike'
PR interval	160 ms
QRS duration	Prolonged (186 ms)
T waves	Normal
QTc interval	Normal (430 ms)

ANSWERS

1. A small pacing 'spike' is seen immediately before each wide QRS complex – this is a ventricular pacing spike. In addition, there is an additional pacing spike visible about 160 ms before most of the QRS complexes – these are the pacemaker signals to the atria which trigger atrial systole. This is **atrioventricular sequential** (or '**dual chamber**') **pacing**.

2. The atrial lead only generates an electrical impulse if the sinoatrial node fails to do so; here, every atrial impulse is pacemaker-activated, according to a preset rate. The ventricular lead only generates an electrical impulse if ventricular contraction does not occur within a fixed time period after the atria have been paced. Here, every ventricular contraction is also pacemaker activated.

3. The patient had episodes of collapse due to complete heart block. As the individual was very active and the ECG showed P waves, a dual chamber pacemaker was implanted. This restores the electrical connection between atria and ventricles, ensuring that atrial and ventricular stimuli are coordinated, avoiding 'pacemaker syndrome'– atrial contraction against an atrioventricular valve closed by asynchronous ventricular contraction. Dual chamber pacing mimics the normal physiological action of the heart.

4. Pacemaker function needs checking a few weeks after implantation and at regular intervals thereafter. 'End of battery life' can be predicted to within a few weeks and unit replacement planned.

COMMENTARY

- The symptoms of complete heart block (dizziness, lack of energy, breathlessness and syncope) are usually relieved by a permanent pacemaker.
- The choice of pacemaker is important. Atrioventricular sequential pacing is preferred if there is any atrial activity, to avoid pacemaker syndrome.
- Pacemakers may be single chamber (pacing the atrium in AAI mode or the ventricle in VVI mode) or dual chamber (pacing both atrium and/or ventricle).

Further reading

Making Sense of the ECG 4th edition: Pacemakers and implantable cardioverter defibrillators, p 209.

CASE 63

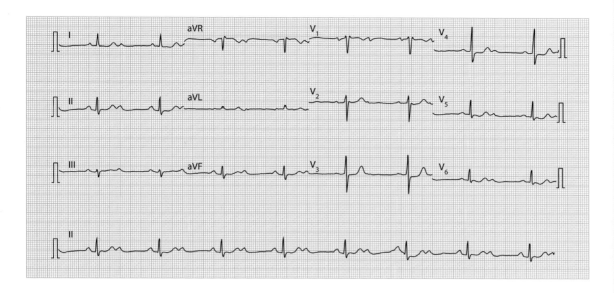

CLINICAL SCENARIO

Female, aged 77 years.

Presenting complaint
Dizzy spells.

History of presenting complaint
Intermittent dizzy spells for one month.

Past medical history
Angina. Diabetes mellitus.

Examination
Pulse: 48/min, regular.

Blood pressure: 140/76.
JVP: not elevated.
Heart sounds: normal.
Chest auscultation: unremarkable.
No peripheral oedema.

Investigations
FBC: Hb 13.4, WCC 7.8, platelets 220.
U&E: Na 141, K 4.6, urea 5.5, creatinine 88.
Thyroid function: normal.
Chest X-ray: normal heart size, clear lung fields.
Echocardiogram: normal cardiac structure and function.

QUESTIONS

1. Describe the appearances seen in this ECG.
2. What arrhythmia is this?
3. How would you manage this arrhythmia?

ECG ANALYSIS

Rate	Atrial – 96/min
	Ventricular – 48/min
Rhythm	Sinus rhythm with second-degree atrioventricular block (2:1)
QRS axis	Normal (+16°)
P waves	Normal
PR interval	Normal for conducted beats (150 ms)
QRS duration	Normal (94 ms)
T waves	Normal
QTc interval	Normal (384 ms)

ANSWERS

1. Every alternate P wave is followed by a QRS complex.
2. Second-degree atrioventricular block (2:1 subtype).
3. Review the patient's medication for any drugs that may cause atrioventricular block (e.g. beta blockers, rate-limiting calcium channel blockers, digoxin). In the absence of a reversible cause, patients with second-degree atrioventricular block (2:1) will usually need permanent pacing and should therefore be referred to a cardiologist.

COMMENTARY

- Second-degree atrioventricular block of the 2:1 subtype means that only every alternate P wave will be conducted via the atrioventricular node. Thus the ventricular (QRS complex) rate will be exactly half of the atrial (P wave) rate.
- Second-degree atrioventricular block is often categorized as Mobitz type 1 or Mobitz type 2, depending upon whether or not the PR interval lengthens before a P wave fails to conduct. However, in 2:1 atrioventricular block it is impossible to say whether the PR interval would have lengthened or not, as there is only one PR interval to measure before the non-conducted P wave occurs. It is therefore impossible to place this into either the Mobtiz type 1 or the Mobitz type 2 category, and so this form of second-degree atrioventricular block is placed in its own category of 2:1 atrioventricular block.

Further reading

Making Sense of the ECG 4th edition: Second-degree atrioventricular block, p 94; 2:1 atrioventricular block, p 96.

Epstein AE, DiMarco JP, Ellenbogen KA *et al.* ACC/AHA/HRS 2008 guidelines for device-based therapy of cardiac rhythm abnormalities. A Report of the American College of Cardiology/American Heart Association task force on practice guidelines (writing committee to revise the ACC/AHA/NASPE 2002 guideline update for implantation of cardiac pacemakers and antiarrhythmia devices). *J Am Coll Cardiol* 2008; **51**: e1–62.

The Task Force on Cardiac Pacing and Resynchronization Therapy of the European Society of Cardiology (ESC). 2013 ESC guidelines on cardiac pacing and cardiac resynchronization therapy. *Eur Heart J* 2013; **34**: 2281–329.

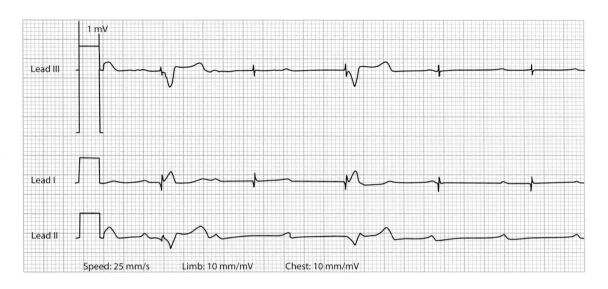

Lead III

Lead I

Lead II

1 mV

Speed: 25 mm/s   Limb: 10 mm/mV   Chest: 10 mm/mV

CLINICAL SCENARIO

Male, aged 83 years.

Presenting complaint
Dizziness.

History of presenting complaint
Recently moved into sheltered accommodation to live near his daughter following his wife's death. Was found collapsed by warden. Seen in the emergency department and found to be extremely bradycardic. No further information available at time of admission.

Past medical history
Prescription in pocket – history of hypertension (on three anti-hypertensive agents). Permanent pacemaker implanted 11 years earlier.

Examination
Pulse: <30/min, irregular.

Blood pressure: 102/68.
JVP: normal.
Heart sounds: normal first and second sound; quiet ejection systolic murmur.
Chest auscultation: a few basal crackles.
No peripheral oedema.

Investigations
FBC: Hb 11.7, WCC 8.1, platelets 178.
U&E: Na 131, K 3.9, urea 12.3, creatinine 221.
Thyroid function: normal.
Troponin I: negative.
Chest X-ray: mild cardiomegaly, early pulmonary congestion.
Echocardiogram: thickened aortic valve with pressure gradient of 22 mmHg. Concentric left ventricular hypertrophy, systolic function moderately impaired (ejection fraction 44 per cent).

QUESTIONS

1. What does this ECG show?
2. What is the mechanism of this?
3. What are the key issues in managing this patient?

ECG ANALYSIS

Rate	<30/min
Rhythm	Pacing spikes with intermittent failure to capture
QRS axis	N/A
P waves	Present, with an atrial rate of 80/min
PR interval	N/A
QRS duration	Prolonged (132 ms)
T waves	N/A
QTc interval	N/A

ANSWERS

1. This rhythm strip shows leads I, II and III. P waves can be seen (particularly clearly in lead II) with an atrial rate of around 80/min. There are also occasional pacing spikes, with a pacing rate of 66/min, but only two of these pacing spikes are followed by QRS complexes. A ventricular pacemaker is therefore trying to pace the ventricles at 66/min, but only intermittently succeeding in doing so. This is therefore underlying complete heart block and **ventricular (VVI) pacing with intermittent failure to capture**.

2. The pacing stimulus is delivered by the pacemaker but the ventricular myocardium fails to depolarize. This can be caused by:
   - displacement of the ventricular lead from its optimal position adjacent to the ventricular myocardium
   - malfunction of the pacing lead (e.g. lead fracture)
   - a change in the pacing threshold (the voltage needed to depolarize the ventricle), as a result of myocardial infarction or ischaemia, electrolyte abnormalities or drug therapy
   - inappropriate programming (inadequate voltage).

3. The underlying cause of the loss of capture needs to be identified and addressed (see above). A chest X-ray will show the position of the pacing lead and whether it has become damaged or dislodged. If the problem is due to a problem with the pacemaker system itself, it may require reprogramming, or repositioning/replacement of the pacing lead.

COMMENTARY

- Pacemaker problems include failures in sensing and failures in pacing.
- **Failure to sense:** the intrinsic intra-cardiac activity is not recognized by the pacemaker because of:
  - inappropriate lead placement
  - lead displacement – usually within a few weeks of pacemaker implantation
  - lead fracture or insulation defect – can occur months or years after implantation; manufacturer will advise if problem occurs with a faulty batch; advise manufacturer if lead fracture identified. Occasionally due to 'twiddler's syndrome' (tendency for the patient to rotate the pacemaker unit itself – avoidable by ensuring the size of the pacemaker's pocket is minimized during wound closure)
  - connector problem – lead connection to pacemaker poor
  - inappropriate programming
  - component failure, e.g. magnetic reed switch jammed (rare).
- **Failure to pace:** a pacing stimulus is not delivered when expected, or a stimulus is delivered but the myocardium does not depolarize. A stimulus will not be delivered with:
  - connector problem – a ratchet screwdriver with preset torque ensures satisfactory attachment of the lead to the pacemaker unit. More of a problem if an 'old style' lead is connected to a 'modern' pacemaker unit
  - lead fracture – this is rare but will trigger a manufacturer's alert
  - pulse generator failure – pacemaker failure is usually due to battery depletion.
- **Oversensing:** Pacemaker detects signals other than those intended (e.g. 'cross talk' between atrial and ventricular components of dual chamber pacemaker); this can usually be electrically 'tuned out' by the cardiac physiologist.

- Lead displacement may occur:
  - early (within 6 weeks) – about 1 per cent of ventricular leads and 4 per cent of atrial leads get displaced
  - late – most commonly affecting the atrial lead.

Further reading

Making Sense of the ECG 4th edition: Pacemakers and implantable cardioverter defibrillators, p 209.

CASE 65

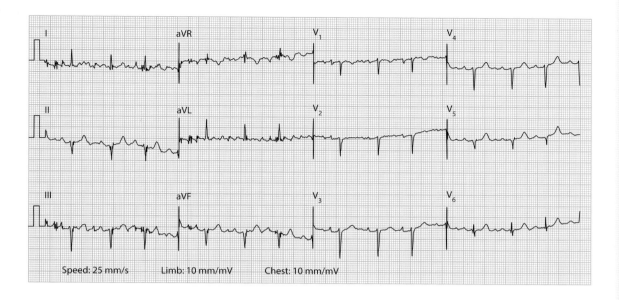

Speed: 25 mm/s   Limb: 10 mm/mV   Chest: 10 mm/mV

CLINICAL SCENARIO

Female, aged 72 years.

Presenting complaint
Exertional breathlessness. Orthopnoea.

History of presenting complaint
One-year history of gradually worsening breathlessness with a reduction in exercise capacity – the patient can now walk only 100 m on level ground. Recent orthopnoea – the patient sleeps with four pillows.

Past medical history
Inferior myocardial infarction 7 years ago. Anteroseptal myocardial infarction 4 years ago. Essential tremor.

Examination
Resting tremor affecting the hands.
Pulse: 90/min, regular.
Blood pressure: 118/74.
JVP: elevated by 3 cm.
Heart sounds: soft (2/6) pan-systolic murmur at apex.
Chest auscultation: bibasal inspiratory crackles. No peripheral oedema.

Investigations
FBC: Hb 11.8, WCC 5.9, platelets 240.
U&E: Na 137, K 4.1, urea 7.7, creatinine 118.
Chest X-ray: moderate cardiomegaly, pulmonary oedema.
Echocardiogram: dilated left ventricle with moderately impaired systolic function (ejection fraction 35 per cent). Mild functional mitral regurgitation.

QUESTIONS

1. What heart rhythm is evident on this ECG?
2. Are there any other ECG findings?
3. What are the likely causes of these findings?

ECG ANALYSIS

Rate	90/min
Rhythm	Sinus rhythm
QRS axis	Normal (−56°)
P waves	Normal
PR interval	Prolonged (205 ms)
QRS duration	Normal (78 ms)
T waves	Normal
QTc interval	Normal (442 ms)

Additional comments

There are inferior Q waves and there is poor R wave progression in leads V1–V5.

ANSWERS

1. Sinus rhythm, which is best appreciated in the chest leads (V1–V6).
2. There are several findings:
   - The baseline in the limb leads is erratic and masks the P waves, making it difficult to discern the underlying rhythm in these leads. The rhythm is seen much more clearly in the chest leads.
   - There are inferior Q waves.
   - There is poor anterior R wave progression (affecting leads V1–V5).
   - There is left axis deviation.
   - There is mild first-degree atrioventricular block (PR interval 205 ms).
3. There are two causes.
   - The erratic baseline is a consequence of the essential tremor, producing musculoskeletal artefact on the ECG recording.
   - Ischaemic heart disease would account for the inferior Q waves (old inferior myocardial infarction), poor anterior R wave progression (old anteroseptal myocardial infarction), left axis deviation (which can be a consequence of inferior myocardial infarction) and mild impairment of atrioventricular conduction.

COMMENTARY

- The ECG records the electrical activity of the heart, but this is not the only source of electrical activity in the body. Skeletal muscle activity is also picked up on the ECG.
- Where possible, patients should lie still during an ECG recording to minimize skeletal muscle artefact, but this is not always possible, particularly if the patient:
  - is uncooperative or agitated
  - is in respiratory distress
  - has a movement disorder.
- The presence of electrical artefact which is much more marked in the limb leads than in the chest leads (as in this example) strongly suggests that skeletal muscle interference from limb movement is the cause.
- The use of signal-averaged ECGs (to 'average out' random electrical artefacts by combining a number of PQRST complexes) can help to reduce the impact of skeletal muscle artefact, particularly during exercise treadmill testing. However, signal-averaged recordings can introduce artefactual changes of their own and so always interpret such recordings with discretion.

Further reading

Making Sense of the ECG 4th edition: Performing an ECG recording p 21; Patient movement, p 205.
Samaniego NC, Morris F, Brady WJ. Electrocardiographic artefact mimicking arrhythmic change on the ECG. *Emerg Med J* 2003; **20**: 356–7.

CASE 66

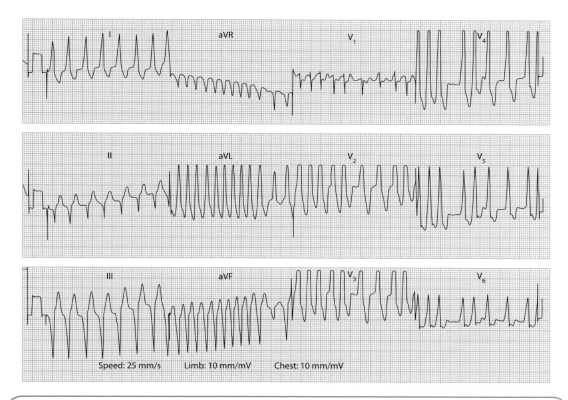

Speed: 25 mm/s   Limb: 10 mm/mV   Chest: 10 mm/mV

CLINICAL SCENARIO

Female, aged 58 years.

Presenting complaint
Palpitations of sudden onset.

History of presenting complaint
Woken from sleep with racing heart beat and breathlessness.

Past medical history
Nil significant.

Examination
Pulse: 228/min, irregularly irregular.
Blood pressure: 110/50.

JVP: not visible.
Heart sounds: hard to assess (tachycardia).
Chest auscultation: fine basal crackles.
No peripheral oedema.

Investigations
FBC: Hb 13.9, WCC 8.1, platelets 233.
U&E: Na 137, K 4.2, urea 5.3, creatinine 88.
Thyroid function: normal.
Troponin I: negative.
Chest X-ray: mild cardiomegaly, early pulmonary congestion.

QUESTIONS

1. What does this ECG show?
2. What is the mechanism of this?
3. What are the key issues in managing this patient?

ECG ANALYSIS

Rate	228/min
Rhythm	Atrial fibrillation with ventricular pre-excitation
QRS axis	Left axis deviation (−49°)
P waves	Not visible
PR interval	N/A
QRS duration	Prolonged (130 ms)
T waves	Inverted in anterolateral leads
QTc interval	Difficult to assess at such high heart rates

ANSWERS

1. This ECG shows irregularly irregular QRS complexes with no discernible P waves, the hallmark of atrial fibrillation. The ventricular rate is very fast. The QRS complexes are somewhat broad and have an odd morphology, not typical of a left or right bundle branch block. This is **atrial fibrillation with ventricular pre-excitation** in Wolff–Parkinson–White (WPW) syndrome.

2. Conduction from atria to ventricles is usually through a single connection involving the atrioventricular node and bundle of His. The ventricles are normally protected from rapid atrial activity by the refractory period of the atrioventricular node. In WPW syndrome, there is an additional *accessory pathway* which conducts electrical activity to the ventricles at a faster rate than the atrioventricular node. If atrial fibrillation develops, most impulses will be conducted via the accessory pathway, so high ventricular rates can be achieved. These beats will contain delta waves as a result of ventricular

pre-excitation (see Case 16). Some impulses will be conducted normally via the atrioventricular node and so normal QRS complexes may be visible at intervals.

3. At very fast heart rates there is a risk of ventricular fibrillation, so consider an urgent cardioversion. Alternatively, you can use a drug that slows conduction through the accessory pathway such as amiodarone or flecainide.

COMMENTARY

- Atrial fibrillation in WPW syndrome can resemble ventricular tachycardia, but AF is irregular whereas ventricular tachycardia is regular.

- In WPW syndrome with atrial fibrillation, the ventricular rate can be very fast due to conduction via the accessory pathway. Blocking the atrioventricular node can paradoxically increase the heart rate even more, by directing all the impulses down the accessory pathway, precipitating ventricular fibrillation. Drugs such as adenosine, beta blockers, verapamil and digoxin must therefore be *avoided* in these patients.

- Urgent cardioversion is the preferred treatment, especially if the patient is hypotensive or in heart failure.

- Patients with WPW syndrome who have had an episode of atrial fibrillation should be referred urgently to a cardiac electrophysiologist for consideration of an accessory pathway ablation procedure.

Further reading

Making Sense of the ECG 4th edition: Wolff–Parkinson–White syndrome, p 69; Atrial fibrillation in Wolff–Parkinson–White syndrome, p 72.

Keating L, Morris FP, Brady WJ. Electrocardiographic features of Wolff-Parkinson-White syndrome. *Emerg Med J* 2003; **20**: 491–3.

CASE 67

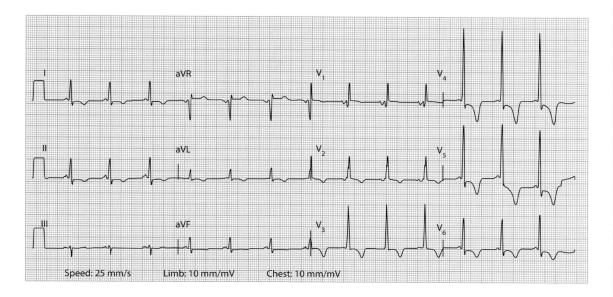

Speed: 25 mm/s   Limb: 10 mm/mV   Chest: 10 mm/mV

CLINICAL SCENARIO

Male, aged 73 years.

Presenting complaint
Breathlessness and peripheral oedema.

History of presenting complaint
Three-month history of progressive breathlessness and peripheral oedema, with a steady fall in exercise capacity.

Past medical history
Hypertension. Chronic obstructive pulmonary disease.

Examination
Patient comfortable at rest but breathless on exertion.

Pulse: 78/min, regular.
Blood pressure: 172/78.
JVP: elevated.
Heart sounds: normal.
Chest auscultation: bilateral expiratory wheeze.
Moderate peripheral oedema.

Investigations
FBC: Hb 10.8, WCC 8.3, platelets 174.
U&E: Na 139, K 4.5, urea 8.2, creatinine 141.
Chest X-ray: pulmonary oedema.
Echocardiogram: moderate hypertrophy of left and right ventricles, and evidence of diastolic dysfunction ('stiff ventricles'). Dilatation of left and right atria.

QUESTIONS

1. What abnormalities are seen on this ECG?
2. How do these abnormalities relate to the echocardiographic findings?
3. What is the likely clinical diagnosis?

ECG ANALYSIS

Rate	78/min
Rhythm	Sinus rhythm
QRS axis	Normal (+30°)
P waves	Normal
PR interval	Borderline short (110 ms)
QRS duration	Normal (90 ms)
T waves	Widespread inversion
QTc interval	Mildly prolonged (456 ms)

Additional comments

There is a dominant R wave in lead V1, and tall R waves in leads V3–V5.

ANSWERS

1. This ECG contains several abnormalities. The main ones are:
   - dominant R waves in the right precordial leads
   - tall R waves in leads V3–V5
   - ST depression and T wave inversion in the anterolateral leads
   - T wave inversion in leads II and aVF.
2. The dominant R waves in the right precordial leads are consistent with right ventricular hypertrophy. The tall R waves in leads V3–V5 are consistent with left ventricular hypertrophy, and the ST segment and T wave abnormalities are consistent with ventricular 'strain' in association with the hypertrophy. The echocardiogram supports these findings, revealing moderate hypertrophy of left and right ventricles.
3. The presence of left ventricular hypertrophy is likely a result of the patient's hypertension. The presence of right ventricular hypertrophy is likely secondary to pulmonary hypertension, which is due to the chronic obstructive pulmonary disease.

COMMENTARY

- Right ventricular hypertrophy causes a 'dominant' R wave (i.e. bigger than the S wave) in the leads that 'look at' the right ventricle, particularly V1. Right ventricular hypertrophy can also cause:
  - right axis deviation
  - deep S waves in leads V5 and V6
  - right bundle branch block (RBBB)
  - ST depression and/or T wave inversion in the right precordial leads (when severe).
- Right ventricular hypertrophy is not the only cause of a positive R wave in lead V1. Other causes include:
  - posterior myocardial infarction
  - Wolff–Parkinson–White syndrome Type A (left sided accessory pathway)
  - dextrocardia.
- Causes of right ventricular hypertrophy include pressure overload on the right ventricle (e.g. pulmonary stenosis, pulmonary hypertension) or hypertrophic cardiomyopathies affecting the right ventricular myocardium. The treatment of right ventricular hypertrophy is that of the underlying cause.

Further reading

Making Sense of the ECG 4th edition: Left ventricular hypertrophy, p 146; Right ventricular hypertrophy, p 147.

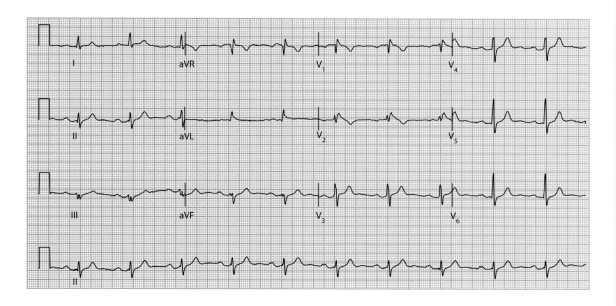

CLINICAL SCENARIO

Male, aged 29 years.

Presenting complaint
Found collapsed at home.

History of presenting complaint
Collapsed without warning at home. On arrival of the paramedics he was found to be in ventricular fibrillation and sinus rhythm was restored following defibrillation.

Past medical history
Nil of note – normally fit and well.

Examination
Pulse: 61/min, regular.
Blood pressure: 126/78.
JVP: not elevated.
Heart sounds: normal.
Chest auscultation: unremarkable.
No peripheral oedema.

Investigations
FBC: Hb 15.4, WCC 6.2, platelets 212.
U&E: Na 142, K 4.3, urea 4.1, creatinine 91.
Troponin I: negative.
Chest X-ray: normal heart size, clear lung fields.
Echocardiogram: normal aortic and mitral valves. Left ventricular function good (ejection fraction 68 per cent).

QUESTIONS

1. What does this ECG show?
2. What is the likely cause of the collapse?
3. What is the underlying mechanism?
4. What are the key issues in managing this patient?

ECG ANALYSIS

Rate	61/min
Rhythm	Sinus rhythm
QRS axis	Normal (+34°)
P waves	Bifid
PR interval	Prolonged (280 ms)
QRS duration	Normal (100 ms)
T waves	Inverted in lead V2
QTc interval	Normal (400 ms)

Additional comments

There is ST segment elevation in leads V1–V3 and a right bundle branch block morphology.

ANSWERS

1. There is ST segment elevation in the right chest leads (V1–V3) and a right bundle branch block (RBBB) morphology – this combination of ECG signs is suggestive of **Brugada syndrome**.

2. In patients with a structurally normal heart but with the ECG characteristics shown above, Brugada syndrome is associated with syncopal or sudden death episodes. The collapse may be due to fast, polymorphic ventricular tachycardia or ventricular fibrillation, usually occurring without warning.

3. Inheritance is autosomal dominant in around 50 per cent of cases and there is an 8:1 male:female ratio. Abnormalities have been identified in the genes coding for ion channels, and in particular the sodium channel gene SCN5A.

4. The diagnosis of Brugada syndrome can be difficult as the ECG changes above may be intermittent or their significance overlooked. ECG abnormalities may be 'unmasked' pharmacologically with flecainide or ajmaline. This particular ECG was recorded during an ajmaline challenge. It is important to exclude electrolyte disorders (hyperkalaemia and hypercalcaemia) and structural heart disease. No drug has been proven effective at preventing arrhythmias or reducing mortality in sudden cardiac death

(SCD) survivors, and so there is a low threshold for using an implantable cardioverter defibrillator (ICD).

COMMENTARY

- Epidemiology:
  - 60 per cent of patients with aborted SCD with typical Brugada ECG have a family history of sudden death or a family with similar ECGs.
  - Brugada syndrome probably accounts for about half of all cases of idiopathic ventricular fibrillation.
  - Incidence probably underestimated: incidence varies with population (26–38/100,000 per year in South East Asia).
  - Recognized worldwide but greatest prevalence in the Far East: 1:2000 of adult Japanese; 1:30,000 in Belgium.
  - Most common cause of sudden death in South Asians under 50 with apparently structurally normal heart.
  - 40 per cent with typical ECG will have a first episode of ventricular tachycardia or sudden death in 3 years, unless asymptomatic with abnormal ECG after drugs.
- Three different ECG patterns have been described in Brugada syndrome. All three have ST segment elevation (≥2 mm elevation of the J point), but vary in other ways:
  - Type 1 has 'coved' ST segment elevation with inverted T waves. The terminal portion of the ST segment gradually descends until it meets the inverted T wave.
  - Type 2 has saddle-shaped ST segment elevation with positive or biphasic T waves. The terminal portion of the ST segment is elevated by ≥1 mm.
  - Type 3 has saddle-shaped ST segment elevation with positive T waves. The terminal portion of the ST segment is elevated by <1 mm.
- Recording the 12-lead ECG with leads V1 and V2 in the second (rather than fourth) intercostal space has been reported to increase the diagnostic sensitivity of the ECG. Some patients require an intravenous challenge with a sodium channel blocking drug (such as flecainide or ajmaline) to

unmask the ECG appearances. This is not helpful in those with a Type 1 ECG, but can help diagnostically in those with Type 2 or 3 ECG appearances. Such a test should only be performed by individuals trained and experienced in the technique.

Further reading

Making Sense of the ECG 4th edition: Brugada syndrome, p 170.

Fitzpatrick AP, Cooper P. Diagnosis and management of patients with blackouts. *Heart* 2006; **92**: 559–68.

Web resource: Brugada Syndrome (www.brugada.org).

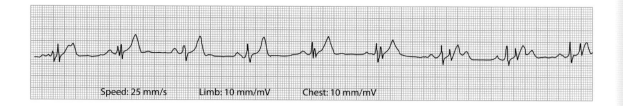

Speed: 25 mm/s   Limb: 10 mm/mV   Chest: 10 mm/mV

CLINICAL SCENARIO

Male, aged 28 years.

Presenting complaint
Palpitations.

History of presenting complaint
Four-month history of episodic palpitations – sudden onset rapid heartbeat, lasting up to 15 min, followed by sudden termination of palpitations. The patient was asymptomatic during the recording of this ECG rhythm strip.

Past medical history
Nil.

Examination
Pulse: 54/min, regular.
Blood pressure: 136/88.
JVP: not elevated.
Heart sounds: normal.
Chest auscultation: unremarkable.
No peripheral oedema.

Investigations
FBC: Hb 14.7, WCC 5.8, platelets 339.
U&E: Na 142, K 5.1, urea 4.5, creatinine 76.
Thyroid function: normal.

QUESTIONS

1. This rhythm strip is taken from a 24-h ambulatory ECG recording – what does it show?
2. What can cause this?
3. What would you do next?

ECG ANALYSIS

Rate	Difficult to assess in view of bizarre rhythm
Rhythm	Bizarre – there appear to be two distinct overlapping rhythms
QRS axis	Unable to assess (single lead)
P waves	Difficult to assess in view of bizarre rhythm
PR interval	Difficult to assess in view of bizarre rhythm
QRS duration	Difficult to assess in view of bizarre rhythm
T waves	Difficult to assess in view of bizarre rhythm
QTc interval	Difficult to assess in view of bizarre rhythm

ANSWERS

1. This is a very odd ECG recording. On close inspection there appear to be two distinct heart rhythms occurring simultaneously, with no obvious correlation between them. In some cases two distinct QRS complexes occur on top of, or close to, each other.
2. In this case, the rhythm strip was made using an old 24-h ECG recorder that used cassette tapes to record the ECG. The cassette tape had been accidentally re-used without the previous recording having been deleted, and so two recordings from different patients ended up on the same cassette tape. When the tape was analyzed, the two recordings appeared simultaneously on one rhythm strip. A similar appearance can be seen in patients who have received a heterotopic 'piggy-back' heart transplant, in which a donor heart is connected to the patient's own heart. Both hearts operate independently, and so an ECG will show two distinct heart rhythms, one from each heart.
3. Discard this recording and arrange a new 24-h ECG recording.

COMMENTARY

- Always consider the possibility of artefact in 'bizarre' ECGs, particularly when they do not correlate with what you know about the patient's clinical details.
- Rare artefactual errors of this kind highlight the importance of taking a careful and structured approach to ECG interpretation, and to ensure that any abnormalities you see can be accounted for.
- This kind of recording error should no longer be possible now that cassette tapes have been superseded by digital recording onto memory cards in ambulatory ECG monitoring.
- In patients with a heterotopic 'piggy-back' heart transplant, a similar 'double ECG' can be seen. In this type of heart transplant, the recipient's heart is left in situ to supplement the function of the donor heart. Heterotopic heart transplants are rarely performed, but may be appropriate if the donor heart is unable to function alone (for example, if the recipient's body size is much greater than that of the donor's, or if the recipient has pulmonary hypertension).

Further reading

Making Sense of the ECG 4th edition: Artefacts on the ECG, p 203.

CASE 70

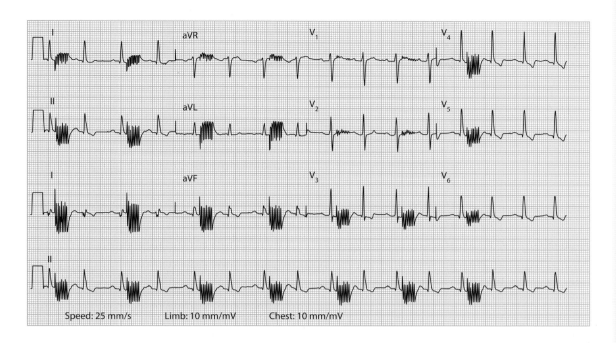

Speed: 25 mm/s   Limb: 10 mm/mV   Chest: 10 mm/mV

CLINICAL SCENARIO

Male, aged 36 years.

Presenting complaint
Breathlessness on exertion.

History of presenting complaint
Patient was fit and well until 12 months earlier. Heart failure had developed after a flu-like illness – viral myocarditis diagnosed. Assessed for cardiac transplant but turned down as had had problems with depression including one (much regretted) suicide attempt. An alternative operation had been offered and performed, and this ECG was recorded post-surgery.

Past medical history
Viral myocarditis.
Depression.

Examination
Pulse: 96/min, regular.
Blood pressure: 108/76.
JVP: not elevated.
Heart sounds: normal.
Chest auscultation: unremarkable.
No peripheral oedema.

Investigations
FBC: Hb 15.9, WCC 6.6, platelets 222.
U&E: Na 143, K 4.1, urea 4.7, creatinine 106.
Thyroid function: normal.
Troponin I: negative.
Chest X-ray: mild cardiomegaly, early pulmonary congestion.
Echocardiogram: moderate mitral regurgitation and dilated left atrium. Left ventricular function severely impaired (ejection fraction 23 per cent).

QUESTIONS

1. What does this ECG show?
2. What operation has this patient undergone?

ECG ANALYSIS

Rate	96/min
Rhythm	Sinus rhythm
QRS axis	Normal (+23°)
P waves	Normal
PR interval	Normal (184 ms)
QRS duration	Normal (110 ms)
T waves	Inverted in inferior and anterolateral leads
QTc interval	Normal (440 ms)

Additional comments

After some of the QRS complexes there is a pacing spike followed by a burst of electrical 'noise' from skeletal muscle.

ANSWERS

1. The ECG shows a normal P wave, PR interval and QRS duration and multiple pacing spikes which occur after many of the QRS complexes. This is the ECG from a patient who has undergone a **dynamic cardiomyoplasty**.
2. This operation, which was sometimes undertaken during the 1980s and 1990s, involved mobilizing the patient's left latissimus dorsi muscle as a pedicle graft, wrapping the free end around the heart and stimulating it to contract in synchrony with cardiac systole. Based on animal and human studies, the benefits of this operation were believed to be due to:
   - a chronic girdling effect due to the wrapping of latissimus dorsi around the heart, resulting in stabilization of the ventricular remodelling process and a decrease in left ventricular dilatation
   - active systolic assistance to decrease myocardial stress.

The operation was performed for patients with heart failure which was symptomatic despite maximal medical treatment. The skeletal muscle had to be 'trained' to work like cardiac muscle – a pacing electrode was placed within the muscle and over a period of weeks stimulated by an impulse generator synchronized with cardiac contraction.

COMMENTARY

- Dynamic cardiomyoplasty was once used as an alternative to cardiac transplantation.
- Perioperative mortality was about 10 per cent.
- 'Muscle transformation' – training the latissimus dorsi muscle by pacing every fourth, third, alternate and finally every cardiac contraction – would take at least eight weeks.
- Trials reported an increase in left ventricular ejection fraction, left ventricular stroke index and stroke work.
- Outcomes were disappointing and the operation was abandoned in the US and UK.

Further reading

Treasure T. Cardiac myoplasty with the latissimus dorsi muscle. *Lancet* 1991; **337**: 1383–4.

Yilmaz MB, Tufekcioglu O, Korkmaz S *et al.* Dynamic cardiomyoplasty: impact of effective pacing. *Int J Cardiol* 2003; **91**: 101–2.

Index